HYBRID STRENGTH
TRAINING

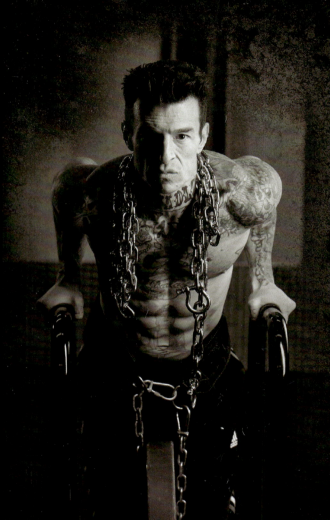

HOW TO GET JACKED AND SHREDDED WITH CALISTHENICS & FREE WEIGHTS

DANNY 🔥 KAVADLO

HYBRID STRENGTH

TRAINING

HOW TO GET JACKED AND SHREDDED WITH CALISTHENICS & FREE WEIGHTS

A Dragon Door Publications, Inc. production
All rights under International and Pan-American Copyright conventions.
Published in the United States by: Dragon Door Publications, Inc.
2999 Yorkton Blvd, Unit 2 • Little Canada, MN 55117
Tel: (651) 487-2180 • Email: support@dragondoor.com • Website: www.dragondoor.com

ISBN 13: 978-1-942812-20-3

This edition first published in October 2021
Printed in China

Book Design: Derek Brigham • www.dbrigham.com • bigd@dbrigham.com

Cover Photo & Photography: M. Nuri Shakoor, Urban Art by Nuri Photography

About the Author Photo: Michael Alago

Additional Photography: Maria Bryk, Eddy Garay, Al Kavadlo, Andrew Lowry, Annie Vo, Danny Weiss

Models: Kristy Agan, Ethan Anderson, Isabella Anderson, Jack Arnow, Wilson Cash Kavadlo, Dave T. Koenig, Errick McAdams, Sean Toomey, Annie Vo

Additional Images: The images on page 2 were drawn by A. Casarin and were originally published in England, 1894 and are in the public domain.

Thanks To: The Kavadlo Family, John Du Cane, Derek Brigham, Paul "Coach" Wade, Al Lewis at Gotham Strength NYC & Mike Anderson.

Special Thanks To: Annie Vo & Wilson Cash Kavadlo for enduring my non-stop company throughout the creation of this project. I could not have done this without you, my family.

Extra Special Thanks To: Everyone who has kept the Dream alive, read one word I've ever written, given me a review, attended PCC, emailed me a question, sent positive feedback, sent negative feedback, liked me, loved me, or even if you've hated me (the haters usually talk more than the lovers!)... Thanks for supporting the cause any way that you can! I AM HERE FOR YOU!

— TABLE OF CONTENTS —

HYBRID STRENGTH TRAINING

F O R E W O R D
By Dan John

One of the hardest things about strength and conditioning coaching, and all areas of personal training, is knitting together all the various tools available to us today. There are probably hundreds of curl machines (just how many ways do we need to get those biceps pumped?) and it's a rare day that someone doesn't show up with another variation of a variation of a variation for the damn lunge.

Danny Kavadlo's new book, **Hybrid Strength Training**, is your step-by-step guide to utilizing barbells, bodyweight, pull-up bars and dip racks to change the way you move and feel. Danny walks us through the basics of basic training. He shows us how to do the most important exercises that every BODY should know and then...

And then he details how to combine these movements into a training system. Danny's work reminds me of how "we" were taught back in the day. Before I become the man yelling at clouds, let me just say that Danny's book reflects the great tradition of strength, physique, and exercise books.

It's not a dissertation on one or two moves that, in total candor, you would be embarrassed to do in a typical gym. Honestly, it's what "we" do... we being coaches and trainers truly interested in improving the lives of our athletes and clients.

Danny's approach to the basics of teaching the movements is sound and simple. There are excellent additional hints sprinkled throughout the chapters on movement and the experienced coach will nod along and then steal the insights for the next training session.

I liked the explanations on the why and how of the book, but what got me really excited was the programming. I would strongly suggest you read and practice the movements before beginning his programs. Having said that, you will have an excellent break-in period for each of his protocols. Danny's sense of humor comes out clearly in the titles of his programs.

As we approach the *Blue Flame* training, I found a bit of joy in discovering that Danny has returned us to the simplicity and logic of the whole-body workout. We balance our week with an upper body day and a lower body day yet come back to circuit training one day a week. Although I might just be an experiment of one (n=1 is the new cool way to say it), but my body reveled in doing this EXACT system decades ago after years of overtraining. (For the record, when you look up the word "overtraining" in the dictionary, you find my picture.)

The standards for the next program, *Red Hot*, mirror what many of us in the field think is an appropriately strong level of lifts for that odd category we call "most of us." Squatting bodyweight and doing five pull ups, as well as reasonable push up and deadlift standards, reflects a vision of common sense.

I like this idea of being asked to establish a standard before moving along to a harder program. None of Danny's standards are crazy, extreme, or mind-bending. But, if you can do them, you should note a change in your physique...and your ability to help people move couches.

Hellyeah! is probably the workout protocol that really ties Danny's vision of "Hybrid Training" together. If you can do the standards of the Hellyeah! program, you really won't have to worry about any gaps in your training or physique. If you get that far, look into Danny's bonus program Deadlift Deathstroke, which is something I think might frighten many of his gentle readers. (Eight sets of deadlifts!!!!)

I want to highlight one thing I always like about Danny's work: he discusses the importance of getting the work in and NOT focusing on the outcome. In my world of coaching performance, I stress "Respect the process." We walk together on this point: if you do the work, follow the program, do the do...you will set yourself up for positive results. Whether it is (or is not) a 315-pound bench or a gold medal often depends on the mysterious workings of the universe. Respect the process.

Danny's suggestions about life and living are common sense. Certainly, these are practical points that we probably heard from grandma, but they are always the first thing I discuss when someone is failing and flailing. I will say his point, "Don't let toxic people in," is something I could use a refresher course on.

I'm honored to call Danny my friend. His impact on my field of strength and conditioning continues to expand daily. This book is part of his legacy.

Enjoy.

—Dan John, author, *Never Let Go*

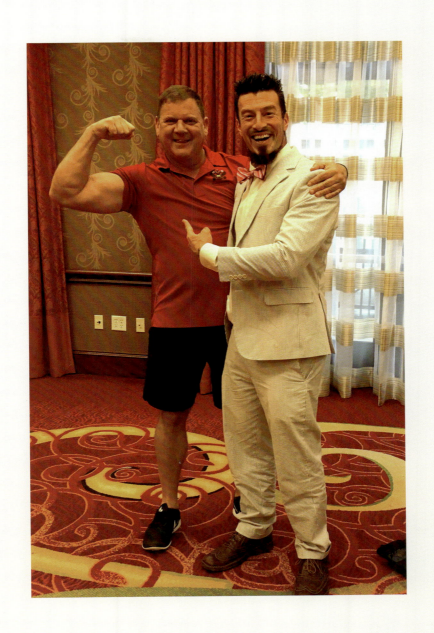

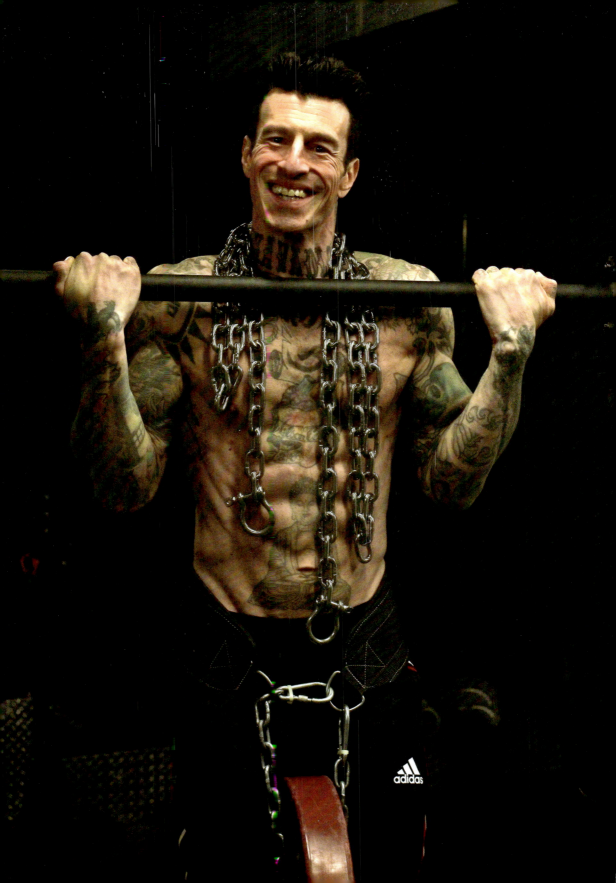

PART I

EXPOSITION

Hello, I'm Danny Kavadlo. I've been working out for over thirty years. Over this time, I've trained extensively in calisthenics, free weights, kettlebells, machines, sandbags and more. As one of New York City's hardest-working trainers for almost two decades, it behooved me to be well versed in multiple modalities of strength training. But even more importantly — as a lifelong student of physical culture — I was constantly seeking out methods and techniques for gaining maximum strength as efficiently and effectively as possible. It made sense to put myself through as many experiences as I could. I'd walk through fire to get strong!

Since 2010, I have been one of the world's most visible proponents of bodyweight training (aka calisthenics). I've published scores of articles about calisthenics and six books, including three #1 Amazon bestsellers. I've taught workshops and certified trainers across the globe, from the US to the UK, Austria to Australia, Sweden to China. And although these certifications are specifically about calisthenics, my own body was built by a combination of calisthenics and weight training.

While I've always emphasised the importance of bodyweight exercise (and still do), I've personally trained in a hybrid style for decades, lifting weights and moving bodyweight side-by-side.

I want to give my clients, my students and myself the best tools for any situation, comprised of the most appropriate exercises for smashing their goals — whether it be calisthenics, free weights or a combination of both. It's a mistake to put a particular ideology ahead of what is best for an individual. My objectives have never been ruled by dogma; they've always been about gains!

It was only after getting more involved with the internet that I became aware of the online rivalry between "calisthenics guys" and "weight lifting bros". Perhaps the gimmicky branding of these two fitness factions, as well as the big-talking nature of the YouTube mob, position them as contrary forces, but they're not. In reality, calisthenics and weight lifting are completely harmonious — waves in the same proverbial ocean. ***Hybrid Strength Training*** is all about eliminating this false distinction in favor of getting the most from our workouts, thus building the greatest body possible.

The strength you get from hybrid training is real strength. In fact, if you were to do an image search of old-time strongmen like Eugen Sandow, Charles Atlas or Steve Reeves— even *Arnold Schwarzenegger* — you'll find them lifting weights and performing bodyweight feats of strength. Hybrid training has a rich history because the two methods complement each other perfectly.

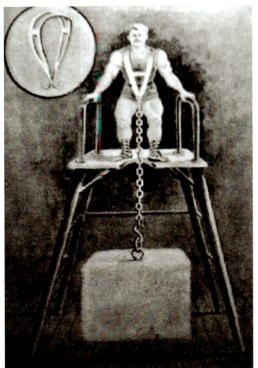 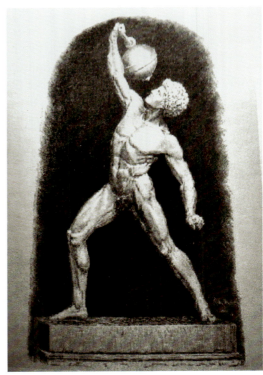

The fusion of external weights and bodyweight training is not new, as illustrated in these drawings by A. Casarin, originally published in 1894.

Efficiency and effectiveness in programming are the keys to unlocking ultimate strength. If we spend our precious energy on ineffective exercises, regardless of our intention, then we are wasting time. We stand to gain the most when we fuse calisthenics and weight training, employing the most effectual exercises from both in order to exhaust the muscles and maximize the value of every workout. Whether you overload your muscles by changing your body's position (as with calisthenics), adding external resistance (as with weight training) or any combination of the two, **you will get results!**

There is an abundance of articles claiming to offer exact bodyweight alternatives to weight training exercises. By the same token there are dozens of apparatuses marketed as simulations of natural movement. These assertions are most likely false on both counts. I choose the words "most likely" because I have not personally read each article or tried every product, otherwise I'd say "definitely".

Both calisthenics and free weights are host to many irreplaceable exercises. For example, even a single leg squat and a hip bridge (both excellent bodyweight exercises), can never replicate a deadlift. Ever. Or vice versa. Yes, several overlapping main muscle groups are recruited for both, but they are different exercises.

The complete truth is that each of these modalities offers its own unique benefits, and we're selling ourselves short if we don't employ them. That's the motivation behind the programs offered in *Hybrid Strength Training.* These programs will get you jacked, shredded and strong. There are three six-week programs included in this manual:

PROGRAM 1 — BLUE FLAME is a beginner to intermediate level program. It consists of progressive weekly workouts so you can familiarize yourself with the basics and beyond. Prepare to blast off from your starting point.

PROGRAM 2 — RED HOT targets the intermediate to advanced level practitioner. It builds upon your starting point, incorporating more exercises and tougher workouts, taking your fitness to new levels.

PROGRAM 3 — HELLYEAH! consists of advanced exercises and programming. This is not for the faint of heart. Prepare to rocket through the stratosphere and get in better shape than you ever thought possible.

Each program concludes with a Self Assessment. This is a chance to test yourself on classic benchmarks of physical strength, so you can properly monitor your progress and see how you measure up.

Come walk through the fire.

WHY CALISTHENICS?

1. **Minimal Equipment** - Calisthenics give the highest yield from the least gear. By manipulating the body's leverage, range of motion and/or muscular emphasis, you can work every muscle in the body, equipment-free (or *equipment-lite*).
2. **Compulsory Creativity** - Having less with which to work compels us to get creative with what we do have. As you will see, a single step or pull-up bar can be used for a multitude of exercises.
3. **Superior Baseline** - A baseline in fundamental calisthenics is necessary before pursuing weight lifting. Period. For example, no one should perform a barbell squat until they are comfortable with a bodyweight squat. You must learn to move yourself before you learn to move an external weight.

CALISTHENICS IS NOT GYMNASTICS!

Although calisthenics and gymnastics have a lot in common, they are not the same. Both employ bodyweight and little else, but gymnastics is a competitive discipline judged by a set of rules, like any other sport or Olympic event. Calisthenics is a style of training, not a competition. Exercises are scalable and practice-oriented as opposed to rigid and goal-oriented. Calisthenics incorporates elements from gymnastics, but they are not the same.

CALISTHENICS GEAR

One of the best aspects of calisthenics training is that you don't need much. In fact, many exercises like push-ups, squats, lunges and sit-ups require no equipment at all! Even when bodyweight exercises call for equipment, the needs are minimal. A pull-up bar and something to step on — maybe some dip bars and a chain — are all you'll need.

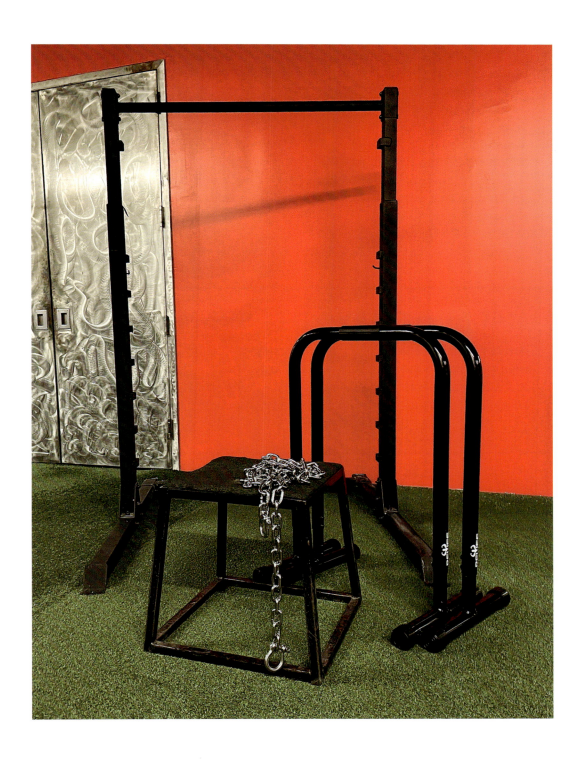

WHY FREE WEIGHTS?

1. **Target Muscles -** Although complete 100% isolation of any muscle is impossible (and arguably undesirable), the nature of training with free weights allows us to target individual muscles and/or muscle groups with greater specificity than other modalities, while still employing our own powers of stability, balance and intramuscular communication.
2. **Simply Scalable Exercises -** To increase the difficulty of a weight lifting exercise, the load can be adjusted by adding or taking away external weight. This is usually much simpler than having to switch to a harder exercise, or learn a new variation, as is the case when no weights are used.
3. **Ability to Go Heavier -** The use of external weight provides the opportunity to lift a greater absolute load than the weight of an individual's own body.

MACHINES ARE NOT FREE WEIGHTS!

Most large workout machines found in gyms swaddle and support your body. By contrast, when you work out with free weights, you rely on yourself for stability and security, not a giant device. When you're not strapped into a machine, you are in control of the weight you lift. You alone keep it steady and evenly distributed, without the use of a sliding track.

FREE WEIGHT GEAR

Most of the primary weight training exercises in this book call for a barbell and a set of weights. Some of the lifts also require a bench or rack. A set of dumbbells will round out your collection. If you choose, kettlebells can be used for many of these exercises too.

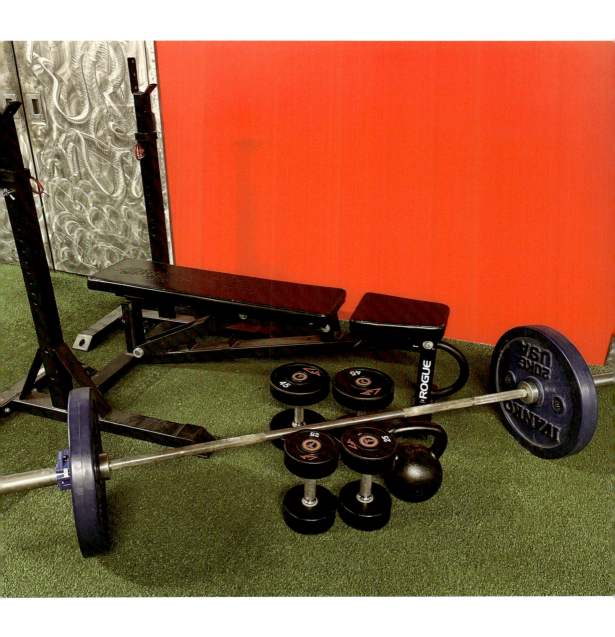

WHY HYBRID TRAINING?

1. **Your Muscles Don't Know the Difference -** *Hybrid Strength Training* refers to the fusion of calisthenics and free weights. This includes weighted calisthenics as well. When you progressively overload your muscles, whether by adjusting the angle of your body as in calisthenics, adding external resistance as in weight training or both, you will get stronger.

2. **Do ALL the Best Exercises -** I know a lot of self-proclaimed "calisthenics guys" who would really benefit from deadlifting. And I know a lot of die-hard "barbell bros" who'd be far better off if they step up their pull-up game. Great exercises are not mutually-exclusive when it comes to getting jacked and shredded.

3. **Freedom from Dogma -** The man who claims to know himself is actually limiting himself. When you choose a program based on results not credo, you strip yourself of self-imposed limitations.

BEST OF BOTH WORLDS

I've often asked my students, *"What do you consider to be strength — the ability to do perfect one-arm push-ups or to bench press 400 lbs?"* The answer, of course, is both. And when seeking strength, we must be open to both. Weight training allows for maximal absolute strength gains, while bodyweight training promotes bodily harmony and relative strength. Employ both to get in the greatest shape of your life.

UNITY

Purposeful division and disdain have no place in the gym (or elsewhere). These various forms of strength training have a lot more in common than apart — all exercise does. So do people.

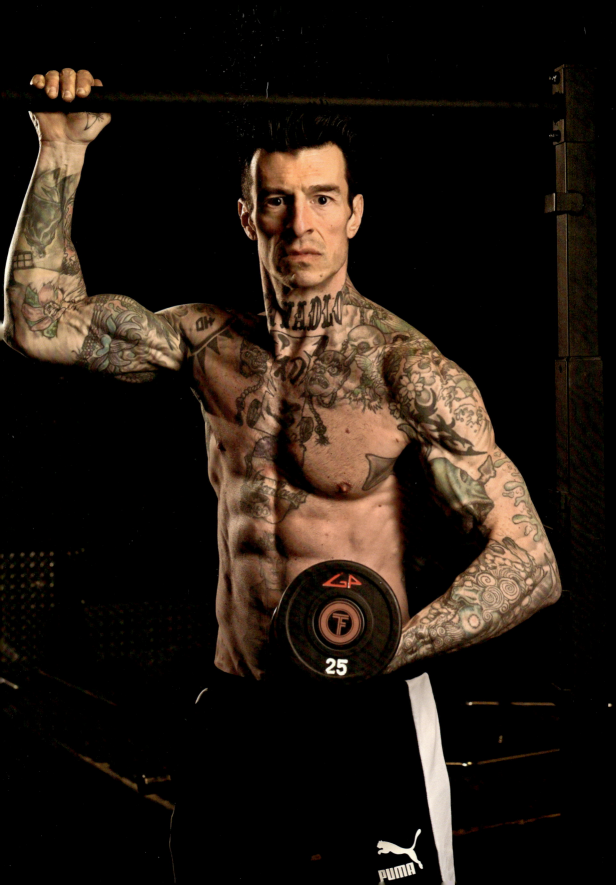

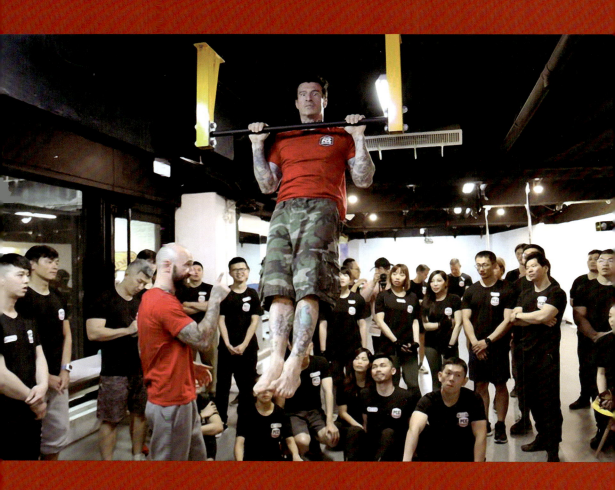

HYBRID STRENGTH TRAINING

PART II

PRIMARY PRINCIPLES

Not everything in or out of the gym affects us all identically. In fact, exercise (as well as other activities) may not even affect the *same person* the same way every time.

Still, there are some overlapping principles that can be universally applied to just about everyone, every time. We all benefit from working out. The better armed we are with information, the more we stand to gain.

Ahead, we address the facts, as well as some of the fiction, about strength training. Be mindful of these concepts and considerations as you exercise. It's one thing to read about training in a book; it's another to experience it.

THE FUNDAMENTALS OF STRENGTH TRAINING

Progressive Overload - Progress in strength training is made by progressive overload. In other words, we get stronger by practicing movement patterns at a low resistance and then over the course of time, increasing that resistance. **Your muscles gradually adapt, growing bigger and stronger.** With free weights, this is accomplished by adding more external weight. With calisthenics (since you can't change your body's weight from set to set), we can alter our leverage or adjust the weight-to-limb ratio. Strength gains cannot be accomplished without progressive overload.

Hypertrophy - This is when your muscles increase in size due to exercise. **This happens when muscles are damaged through outside stressors (exercise) — then through nutrition, rest and recovery, they repair and grow.** Think about it: Just like you get stronger from stressful situations, so do your muscles. You've been through some tough stuff, right? And you're probably stronger for it. Your muscles are the same way. Like you, they have to go through some trauma so they can grow and become more resilient.

Form - The notion of "form" refers to the technique of performing an exercise properly and safely. Exercise is one of the few things we do that is purposely difficult. Usually, we strive to make all life's tasks as easy as possible. But with working out, this is not conducive to results. We get more out of exercise if we're challenged. Form does not exist for the sake of having an arbitrary set of rules. **Form exists so that you can get the very most out of every exercise you do.** Proper form can also help in preventing injury, but in reality, workout injuries are rare. Sure, employing good form will keep you safe, but it will also make you stronger.

Range of Motion - If you want to possess strength at every angle (and for your muscles to get bigger, stronger and better defined), then perform the full range of motion (ROM) of every repetition. **Start at the beginning position and, in a deliberate fashion, perform the entire exercise on both the concentric and eccentric phases to the fullest expression.** It's important to prioritize quality over quantity.

Full Body Engagement - Maintaining muscular tension throughout your entire body during exercise contributes to strength, clear-mindedness and anatomical awareness. While the exercises in this book are separated into categories based on the primary muscles recruited, make no mistake: I want you to maintain a tense, fully-engaged body for the complete execution of every single exercise. Don't relax in the negative phase or disengage your muscles at the end of a repetition. **Engage all your muscles — not just the primary movers — the whole time**. So dig your heels and toes into the ground, tighten those glutes, engage your lats and brace your abs. Squeeze with your hands and feet. This will help facilitate everything, including greater muscle recruitment, increased muscle growth and larger energy expenditure.

Time Under Tension - The phrase "time under tension" refers to how long a muscle (or group of muscles) is under stress. A greater time under tension overloads the muscle by increasing the duration, rather than load, of an exercise. **This can be achieved by slowing down the speed at which you perform the exercise.** You can even pause for a moment at the top, bottom or middle of a repetition.

The Basics - There are almost endless variations of every exercise in existence. **The exercises included in this manual are the ones I use because they work, not because they're trendy.** In fact, quite the opposite: because they're timeless. All beginners need to start with the basics. Advanced practitioners need to continue with the basics. To be fair, there will be times where it is appropriate to incorporate more esoteric exercises, such as sports specific training, corrective rehabilitation or to learn a particular move, but this is not the case most of the time.

TRAIN LARGE MOVEMENTS FIRST...

It is important to train the larger exercises early in the workout. They expend more energy, incorporate larger muscle groups and demand the greatest effort. **Movement patterns such as *squats*, *deadlifts*, and *pull-ups*, for example, should usually be performed towards the beginning of a workout.**

...THEN TRAIN SECONDARY ONES

This book includes over one hundred exercises and alternatives, including supplementary movements like *lateral raises, curls* and *sit-ups*. These are all very fine exercises, however I'd like to be clear that if you do not include the large movement patterns in a program, then you are not using your time to the best of your ability. **Secondary exercises are intended to supplement the primary ones, not replace them, so do them later in the workout.** They are important and have their place (as detailed in their descriptions and in the programming section of this book), but only if you're training the primary moves.

STRENGTH DEFINED

Strength comes in many forms. When I talk about the strength you gain from hybrid training, I am referring to physical strength in the following ways:

Relative Strength - How strong you are relative to your size and mass.

It's great to be big and strong, but if you cannot navigate your own body, whatever your size, then you are missing out on the big picture. It's been said that calisthenics is "the great equalizer" of strength training, meaning it is a true indicator of pound-for-pound power. With calisthenics, the small guys can compete with the big guys on a level (and arguably favorable) playing field.

Absolute Strength - Maximum force you can exert regardless of your size.

A counter argument to the "great equalizer" statement above is that if one is small and light, but cannot move a heavy external load, then all the relative strength in the world won't amount to much. Generally speaking, a larger person can move more external weight, compared to a similarly proportioned, but smaller individual. This is "The Flea/Elephant" argument. A flea can pull over 100,000 times its own weight, which is about 1 gram, whereas an elephant can carry only 1 to 1.5 times its bodyweight, but that is up to 6,000 kg.

Physiological Strength - Mind/muscle connection.

I use the term "connection" loosely because the mind and muscle are more than connected — they're one and the same. While generally weight training promotes more absolute strength, and calisthenics leans toward relative strength, in both cases, we always want our body to work as one cohesive unit. The rehearsal of physical movement patterns builds physiological, neuro-muscular strength.

Strength Endurance - How long your muscles can perform.

Honestly, there is a much greater overlap between raw strength (relative and absolute) and strength endurance than is often postulated. When we train hard and push ourselves, our muscles increase in both strength and endurance, not to mention mass. And having greater muscular endurance sets us up for greater strength gains down the road.

Complete Strength - More than physical strength.

Mental health, emotional wellness and individual spirit are all components of complete strength. They are never to be ignored when seeking health. It's a fact that physical exercise stimulates brain activity, improves memory and releases endorphins. The positivity and energy we feel after a workout transcends the physical. While we must pursue cerebral, emotional and artistic endeavors, strength training also provides food for the soul.

EVERYBODY NEEDS STRENGTH TRAINING!   HERE'S WHY:

- Greater Strength
- Increased Muscle Mass
- Faster Metabolism
- Lower Body Fat
- Controlled Blood Sugar Levels
- Heightened Libido
- Greater Cardiovascular Health
- Stronger Bones
- Healthier Joints & Connective Tissue
- Improved Mobility
- Better Posture
- Increased Confidence
- Better Sex
- Deeper Sleep
- Improved Athletic Performance
- More Attractive Appearance
- Easier Stress Management
- Clearer Mind
- Greater Appreciation for Hard Work
- Lower Risk of Injury
- Longer Life

FITNESS MYTHS DEBUNKED!

Now that we've discussed the facts about strength training, it's time to dispel some of the fiction. There's always been falsehood and deception in the fitness department, but these days, it's worse than ever. It's not just equipment manufacturers and chain gyms who profit by misleading. Self-proclaimed gurus make all sorts of unfounded claims from their parents' basement. With the right media design and a following to back them up, many can even appear legit. But appearances have been known to deceive.

Don't believe the hype.

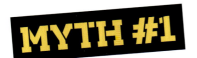

THE BEST PROGRAM FOR EVERYONE

As much as I'd like to tell you that you're holding the best program for everyone in your hands right now, I cannot. The truth is that there is no best program for everyone. If someone is looking to increase their running speed but not gain strength, then this is not the book for them. If you're in search of corrective rehab exercises, agility drills, MMA or Zumba, then there are better resources. If your goal is to make the greatest possible strength gains, become functionally sound and look better with your clothes off, then, *YES, **Hybrid Strength Training*** is for you. And still, I encourage you to make any alterations to this program (or any other) that are relevant and appropriate. People progress differently from one another, sometimes in unexpected ways, even within the same program. Let's acknowledge and celebrate our differences, not pretend they don't exist.

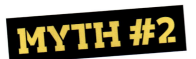

INSTANT TRANSFORMATIONS

When Ernest Hemmingway was asked how he went broke, he famously replied "Gradually, then suddenly." That's how we get out of shape too. It's a slow, creeping process... Until it's not. Falling out of fitness often feels sudden to the one going through it, but it rarely is. The descent into poor health is generally years in the making. So why do so many people think they can turn it around quickly?

Getting in shape is a process that demands hours of real effort, sustained for weeks, months, even years. The so-called "instant" transformations and before and after photos you see in magazines, advertisements and on the internet are fake. These bogus boasts are intended to trick you, but there are no shortcuts. Change takes time and effort. That is part of what makes working out valuable. You can't buy it, hack it, find it or steal it. You must put in the work.

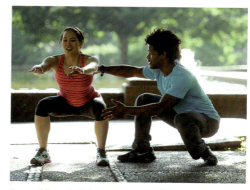

Some things in this world must still be earned.

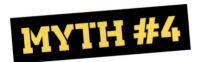

MYTH #3

IT'S EASY TO GET IN SHAPE

If getting in shape were easy, there wouldn't be an obesity epidemic and humankind would not be getting weaker every generation. In an effort to make life effortless, modern humanity has sought to eliminate almost all physically difficult tasks in our day-to-day lives. We've grown deconditioned. Consequently, many have forgotten — or never knew — that exposure to difficult situations is good for us! That's how we (and our muscles) get stronger. And that's why if your workout is easy, then you need to work harder.

Full disclosure: when one is brand new to exercise, almost any muscle stimulation will promote some change — it's the difference between doing nothing and doing anything. But these beginner gains level off over time. Ultimately, there is a direct correlation between the effort you put forth and the results you get.

MYTH #4

SPOT REDUCTION OF BODY FAT

Targeting a particular part of the body such as the belly, arms or butt will not reduce the fat specifically in that area. It doesn't work that way.

We metabolize stored body fat when we expend more energy (through exercise and other activities) than we consume (through food and drink). Therefore, all exercise can potentially reduce fat to some degree. However, this fat comes from many places, not necessarily the target areas. It is unpredictable. Zoning in on a fatty area will sculpt and build the muscle underneath the fat, but fat loss is achieved mostly through diet.

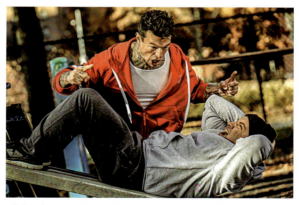

All the sit-ups in the world will not target belly fat.

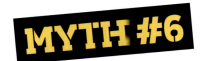

SUPPLEMENTS

A balanced diet, rich in fruits, vegetables and lean protein will give your body a lot more of what it needs than the powders, pills and promises pushed by an all-too-often uncaring industry. Nutrition is better when it comes directly from the source. As an advocate of simple nutrition and an appreciator of delicious foods, it's my duty to point out that dietary supplements (even the ones that claim to be high quality — which is all of them) are simply super-processed food derivatives with excellent marketing. I generally do not recommend supplements for anybody unless they are in a medical deficiency, and even then I'm guarded. In other words, if you're anemic, maybe you could use an iron supplement, but a better approach in most cases would be to eat more iron-rich foods.

On a related note, we do not need as much protein — even when building muscle — as supplement manufacturers claim. I've seen recommendations of up to 2 grams of protein per 1 pound of bodyweight every day, which is insane. Marketing aside, men can build lean muscle mass with fewer than 100 grams of protein a day, and women can with even less (depending on body mass, metabolic rate and genetics). Rather than measuring grams and washing shakers all day, I suggest simply eating protein and fiber with every meal. You do not need a scale. For the record I have not consumed any supplements (protein, creatine or even multivitamins) in almost two decades. Just lots of good food and water.

MYTH #6

CARDIO FOR WEIGHT LOSS

Because cardiovascular exercise is often associated with a high expenditure of energy, many folks conclude that it's best for weight loss. False. Strength training is better for weight loss than cardio every single time. When you synthesize a leaner, more muscular body, your base metabolic rate and daily energy demands increase. By changing your body composition with strength training, you will burn more body fat. But as wonderful as strength training is for weight loss, there is something that works even better: the food you choose to eat. You cannot train your way out of a poor diet.

High Risk of Injury

This fearful falsehood is not only perpetuated by the media, but also by the fitness industry itself. (They'll usually have a new safety product to sell you.) Sure, anyone who trains has the potential to get injured. The same is true for people who don't train. The fact is that working out is healthier and safer, with a lower risk of injury, than *not* working out. It makes you stronger, denser, leaner and more agile, with better circulation, blood flow and endocrine levels, so you're less prone to injury and even illness.

I've been working out for over 30 years and I've never suffered more than temporary discomfort from even my most grueling workouts. This is because I pay attention to my form and to the environment around me. Mindful training is safe training. Careless training has no place. Be present and you'll be bulletproof.

Women Get Bulky if They Lift

Actually the opposite is true. Lifting helps women get leaner. In general, women have a more *difficult* time building muscle than men. This is because of the intrinsic physiological differences between women and men. Women do not manufacture the testosterone needed to synthesize huge muscles without hormonal supplementation. To be fair, men aren't going to unintentionally bulk up either. Getting big from lifting is a great effort, consisting of a multitude of decisions about diet, sleep, stressors and lifestyle—plus the workouts. Putting on muscle does not happen accidentally. Most of the time when women or men get bulky, it's from eating too much.

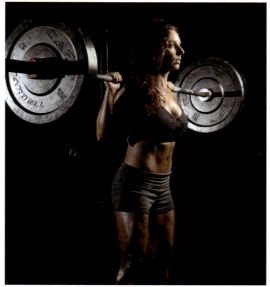

Fun Fact: Women do NOT get huge if they lift.

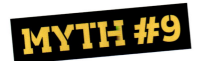

NEW INNOVATIONS

There will always be fly-by-night fitness fads and everyone has something to sell. But you know me: I believe low tech items like a pull-up bar and some weights are the most complicated gear you need. Strength training really hasn't changed much over the years, and neither has the equipment, so don't be swindled. To quote **Arnold's Bodybuilding for Men** (1980): "There are a lot of manufacturers trying to cash in on the national craze for exercise and fitness with devices and springs and levers and chrome doodads that are supposed to help you get in shape. For anyone really serious about training, these things are a waste of money." There you have it.

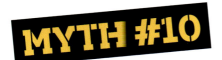

THE AGING PROCESS

A more appropriate title would be the "*I stopped taking care of myself a long time ago*" process. People don't get weaker, sicker or sexually dried out because they age. It happens because they go a really, really long time without taking care of themselves. Decisions like not exercising, overmedicating, not sleeping enough and sitting all day are far more dangerous than the passage of time. Someone who's had these habits for twenty years and has slowly fallen off the deep end will often blame the twenty years but not the habits.

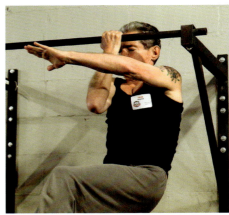

The immortal Jack Arnow performing a one arm chin-up at age 75.

Barring injury or extreme disability, we are all capable of great health until an advanced age. As long as we stimulate ourselves with exercise, books, creative endeavors and action, then the so-called aging process is just chronological wordplay. Of course your body changes as it ages. I would never deny that. But the few negative effects (slower metabolism, joint sensitivity, declining vision) are easily dealt with (eat a little less, work on mobility, wear glasses). I have known many people who have gotten in the best shape of their lives in their 50's, 60's and 70's.

TRUSTING YOUR INSTINCTS

When starting a fitness program or taking workout advice in general, one should evaluate the merit, track record and attitude of any so-called expert, myself included, and use these findings to determine who (or what) is most appropriate to work with.

I used to think it was odd how when it came to exercise, typically confident and self-assured people would become insecure and confused, often second guessing their own common sense. Yet upon reflection, it's actually rather understandable: much of the fitness industry and media deliberately seek to overcomplicate things. They want to mystify and confuse.

Shock and awe.

Then sell you stuff.

But fitness is not as complicated as many credentialed "authorities" would have you believe.

The "appeal to authority" *(argumentum ad verecundiam)* says that for a premise to hold water, the speaker must have the credential of my choosing from the institution of my choice. It's rubbish. Rather than reviewing evidence, proponents of this argument accept the claims of a chosen authority to be true, with or without any real affirmation to support it.

That works for some, but for me, it's not about degrees or certifications. It's about having a successful track record and good vibe. Credentials often mean nothing when it comes to fitness. I know personal trainers who dropped out of 8th grade with more knowledge, wisdom and expertise than others I've known with advanced degrees. True story.

The same can be said of many social media influencers. But rather than use post-nominal letters to advertise their merit, the influencer employs numbers to show how many followers enjoy their cool quotes and pics. For clarity, of course advanced degrees and a large media following can, and often do, correlate with legitimate expertise. However, these traits don't necessarily translate to ability.

Question everything.

If someone suggests an exercise, program, diet or remedy, and it doesn't make sense to you personally, then ask why. If a workout or prescription brings pain, but the video you're watching or personality you follow says to do it anyway, who do you trust? I hope your instincts. You have them for a reason. Pain receptors too.

On that note, it is important to distinguish the difference between pain and discomfort. As we discussed in the previous chapter, we must put ourselves through hardship in order to grow, both in and out of the gym. Your muscles, like you, will never achieve anything great without being challenged. But the pain and discomfort are not the same.

When I say "discomfort" I mean the physical unease that can temporarily occur during or after your workout. This can be in the form of muscular stress, minor aching of the connective tissues or even the delayed onset muscular soreness (DOMS) that may take place days after a training session.

I often enjoy this discomfort. I earned it.

"Pain", by contrast, is sharp and shooting. While discomfort (even when in the form of major soreness) is often a dull, throbbing pulse, pain is more intense and usually pinpoint-able to one single, exact spot. Pain is not enjoyable. It is your nervous system instinctively signaling to your body that you are in potential harm. In that case, it's time to stop and reevaluate. Serious injuries in the gym are generally rare, in part because savvy lifters listen to the signals their bodies give them. If you experience any severe pain or discomfort, or if it goes on for more than a few days, then medical intervention may be needed.

Remember that no matter your goals, program, trainer or coach, no one knows your body better than you. The better you know yourself, the more you will get out of training. The more years you train, the better you'll know yourself.

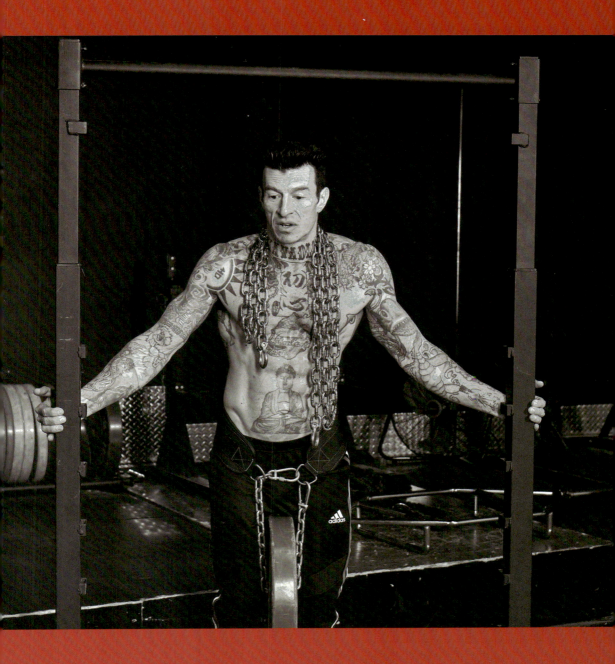

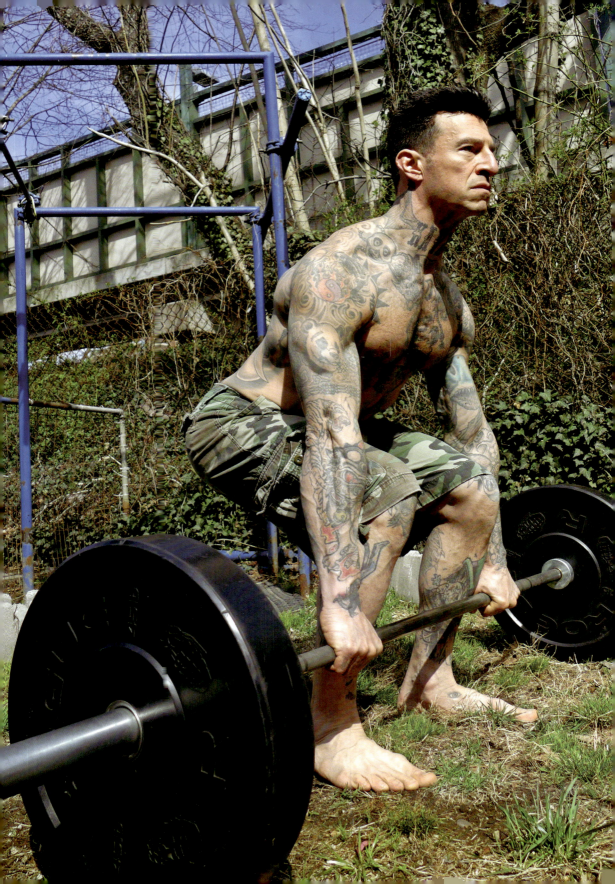

PART III

EXERCISES

The exercises that follow are broken down into six categories based on the primary body part being trained: Legs, Chest, Back, Shoulders, Arms and Abs.

Each exercise is explained with a brief overview, an easy to follow 3-step description and "Trainer Talk", which consists of my personal tips, techniques and observations. I've also included a list of the primary and secondary muscles recruited for each exercise. Some exercises recruit many muscle groups and are therefore impossible to place in one single category. In these cases, this is notated in the description.

No matter what body part you're training, do your best to keep all your muscles flexed and fully-engaged. In order to get as much as you can from every workout, make sure you review the *Fundamentals of Strength Training* beginning on page 11 before moving forward.

What lies ahead are all time-tested exercises, each with a rich history built by champion weightlifters, calisthenics superstars, elite bodybuilders and old school strongmen. Nothing fancy. Just real exercises that work, so you can get jacked, shredded and strong!

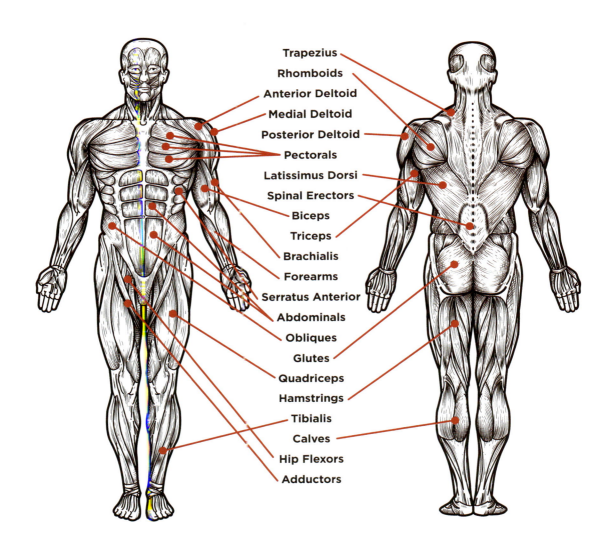

Trapezius

Rhomboids

Anterior Deltoid

Medial Deltoid

Posterior Deltoid

Pectorals

Latissimus Dorsi

Spinal Erectors

Biceps

Triceps

Brachialis

Forearms

Serratus Anterior

Abdominals

Obliques

Glutes

Quadriceps

Hamstrings

Tibialis

Calves

Hip Flexors

Adductors

LEGS

1. Bodyweight Squat
2. Goblet Squat
3. Barbell Squat
4. Bodyweight Split Squat
5. Weighted Split Squat
6. Barbell Split Squat
7. Bodyweight Lunge
8. Weighted Lunge
9. Barbell Lunge
10. Bulgarian Split Squat
11. Weighted Bulgarian Split Squat
12. One Leg Squat
13. Weighted One Leg Squat
14. Hip Bridge
15. One Leg Hip Bridge
16. Deadlift
17. Romanian Deadlift
18. Trap Bar Deadlift
19. Leg Stretches

BODYWEIGHT SQUAT

The squat is the foundational lower body exercise, as well as one of the most important human movement patterns. The bodyweight squat is a prerequisite to any type of weighted squat.

1 - Stand with your feet approximately shoulder width apart.

2 - Reach your arms forward and bend your hips, knees and ankles, lowering yourself down until your thighs come in contact with your calves. Keep your heels flat and your chest up.

3 - Drive your heels down and extend your hips forward simultaneously to return to the starting position.

Trainer Talk: A wider foot position places greater emphasis on the adductors. A narrower foot position places greater emphasis on the quadriceps.

Primary Muscles: Quadriceps, hamstrings, glutes, spinal erectors.

Secondary Muscles: Hip flexors, abdominals, calves.

CAUTION! With bodyweight squats, and all squats, keep your chest up and avoid rounding your upper spine. Make sure your knees track in line with your toes and don't cave in or point out.

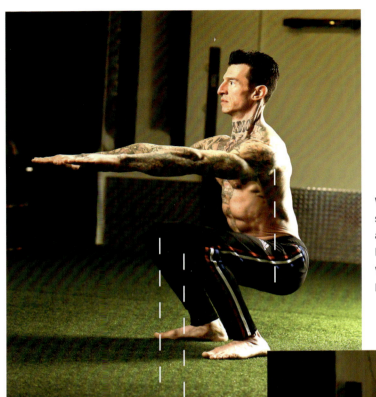

With bodyweight squats, and all squats, keep your chest up and avoid rounding your upper spine. Make sure your knees track in line with your toes and don't cave in or point out.

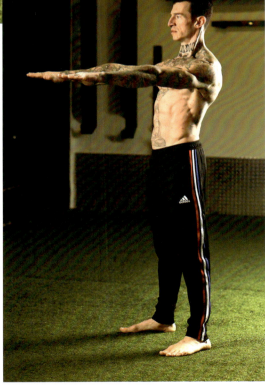

HYBRID STRENGTH TRAINING

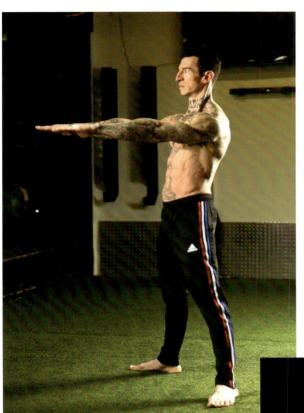

A wider foot position places greater emphasis on the adductors.

A narrower foot position places greater emphasis on the quadriceps. Make sure that your toes and your knees point in the same direction.

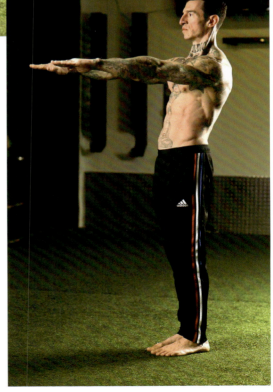

Goblet Squat

Performing goblet squats is a fantastic way to transition from bodyweight squats to barbell squats. The unique position of the weight compels the practitioner to keep their chest up and shoulder blades depressed.

1 - Hold a kettlebell or dumbbell against your chest with both hands, and stand with your feet approximately shoulder width apart.

2 - Squeeze the weight tightly and bend your hips, knees and ankles, lowering yourself down until your thighs come in contact with your calves. Keep your heels flat and your chest up. Your elbows may touch the inside of your thighs.

3 - Drive your heels down and extend your hips forward simultaneously to return to the starting position.

Trainer Talk: Use the weight of the kettlebell to guide your hips down into the bottom position.

Primary Muscles: Quadriceps, hamstrings, glutes, spinal erectors, rhomboids.

Secondary Muscles: Hip flexors, abdominals, calves.

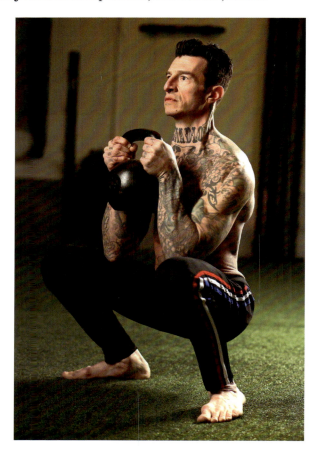

BARBELL SQUAT

The barbell squat is one of the three main powerlifting exercises, and is arguably the most important lift.

1 - Get under the racked barbell so that it rests on your traps, just above your posterior deltoids. Grasp the bar tightly with your chest up, and your feet approximately shoulder width apart. Step back and remove the bar from the rack.

2 - Bend your hips, knees and ankles, lowering yourself down until the tops of your thighs are parallel to the ground. If you are able, lower down until your hamstrings come in contact with your calves. Keep your heels flat on the ground and your chest up.

3 - Drive your heels down and extend your hips forward to return to the starting position.

Trainer Talk: The bodyweight squat is a prerequisite to barbell squats. As with the bodyweight squat, you may experiment with different foot positions; just make sure that your toes and your knees point in the same direction to avoid any shearing.

Primary Muscles: Quadriceps, hamstrings, glutes, spinal erectors.

Secondary Muscles: Hip flexors, abdominals, calves.

CAUTION! I recommend doing an unloaded set with just the barbell to warm up before adding any weight, every time, no matter how strong you are. With bodyweight squats, and all squats, keep your chest up and don't allow your back to round forward. Use a spotter for heavy weight.

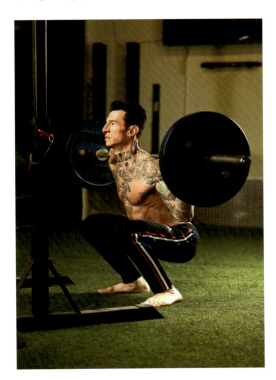
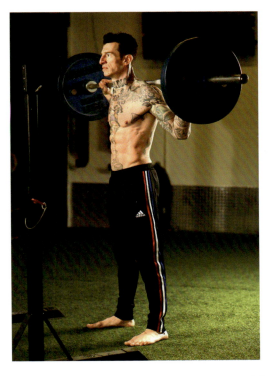

PROTECT YOUR NECK

The barbell should rest on your trapezius, just above your posterior deltoids. Although there is some leeway regarding how high or low it may be placed, the bar should never be on your neck.

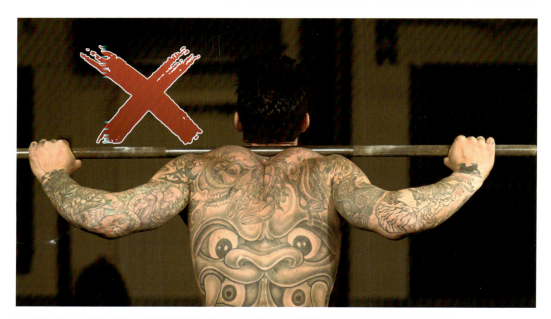

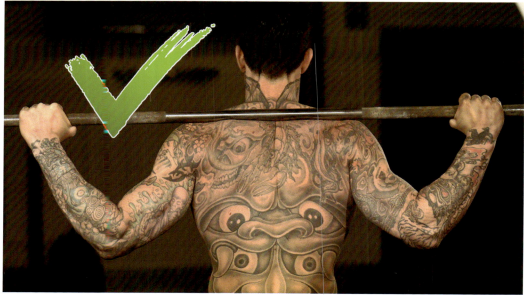

HYBRID STRENGTH TRAINING

FRONT SQUAT RACK POSITION

Barbell squats, split squats and lunges can be performed in a front squat position. In doing so, the exercise becomes more quadriceps dominant than a traditional barbell back position.

Start with your hands approximately shoulder width, bent at the elbow, with your palms facing up. As you approach the bar, press your chest toward it, and rotate your elbows forward. The bar should rest above your chest, snug against your windpipe, across your collarbone. Raise your chest and keep your elbows as high as you can. Step back to unrack the bar.

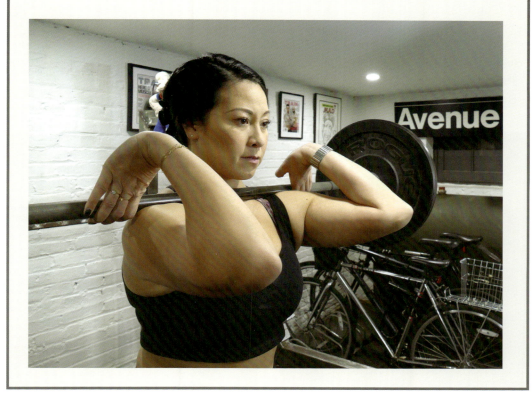

Bodyweight Split Squat

This exercise is asymmetrical in that each leg is doing something different. It is important to train each side evenly.

1 - Stand up straight with your feet approximately shoulder width apart, then take a big step forward with one foot.

2 - Keep your chest up and lower yourself down, bending both knees to approximately 90°. Keep your entire front foot on the ground, while allowing your rear heel to come up. Do not let your rear knee touch the ground.

3 - Pause briefly at the bottom before returning to the top position. Complete your set in its entirety and then repeat on the opposite side.

Trainer Talk: Both legs play a role regardless of which foot is forward. The front foot drives with the heel and the rear foot pushes off with the ball of the foot and toes.

Primary Muscles: Quadriceps, hamstrings, glutes.

Secondary Muscles: Calves, tibialis.

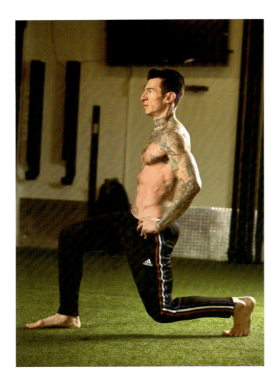
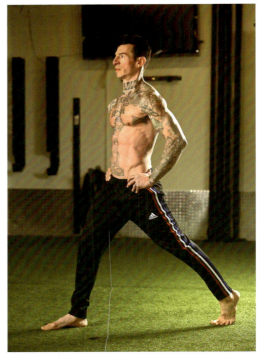

WEIGHTED SPLIT SQUAT

Adding external resistance to this bodyweight classic is a fantastic way to train harder, employ more of your core and trigger greater muscular growth, without having to incorporate a different movement pattern.

1 - Stand up straight with a dumbbell or kettlebell in each hand and your feet approximately shoulder width apart, then take a big step forward with one foot.

2 - Keep your chest up and lower yourself down, bending both knees to approximately 90°. Keep your entire front foot on the ground, while allowing your rear heel to come up. Do not let your rear knee touch the ground.

3 - Pause briefly at the bottom before returning to the top position. Complete your set in its entirety and then repeat on the opposite side.

Trainer Talk: Be careful that you do not pitch your chest forward when performing weighted split squats. The weight, along with your upper body, should descend straight down toward the ground. Maintain control at all times.

Primary Muscles: Quadriceps, hamstrings, glutes.

Secondary Muscles: Calves, tibialis.

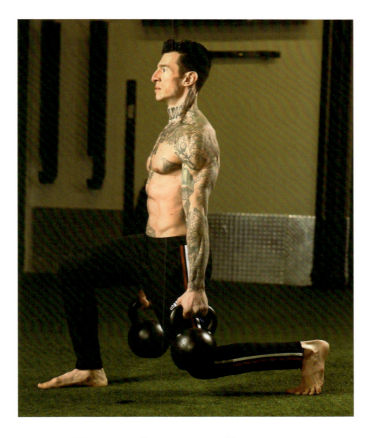

BARBELL SPLIT SQUAT

Holding the barbell on your back places greater demand on your traps, back and shoulders. Barbell split squats require a tremendous amount of abdominal and low back recruitment for stability.

1 - Get under the racked barbell so that it rests on your traps, just above your posterior deltoids. Grasp the bar tightly with your chest up, and your feet approximately shoulder width apart. Step back and remove the bar from the rack. Take a big step forward with one foot.

2 - Keep your chest up and lower yourself down, bending both knees to approximately 90°. Keep your entire front foot on the ground, while allowing your rear heel to come up. Do not let your rear knee touch the ground.

3 - Pause briefly at the bottom before returning to the top position. Complete your set in its entirety and then repeat on the opposite side.

Trainer Talk: The weight of the barbell, along with your upper body, should descend straight down toward the ground. Maintain control at all times.

Primary Muscles: Quadriceps, hamstrings, glutes.

Secondary Muscles: Calves, tibialis.

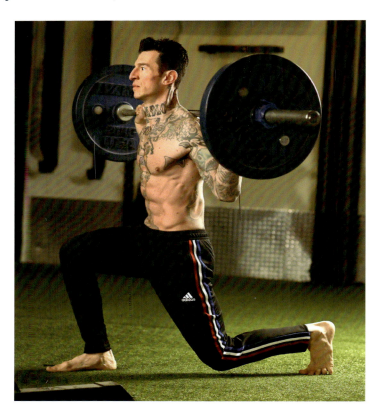

Bodyweight Lunge

Balance is a key component in lunges, as they introduce a dynamic element. Take each step slowly.

1 - Stand up straight with your feet approximately shoulder width apart, then take a big step back with one leg.

2 - Keep your entire front foot on the ground, while allowing your rear heel to come up. Keep your chest up and lower yourself down, bending both knees to approximately 90°. Do not let your rear knee touch the ground.

3 - Drive your front heel and rear toe into the ground to bring your rear leg forward and your feet together again. Alternate sides between repetitions.

Trainer Talk: Lunges can also be done in a walking pattern, where you continually step forward from rep to rep.

Primary Muscles: Quadriceps, hamstrings, glutes.

Secondary Muscles: Calves, tibialis.

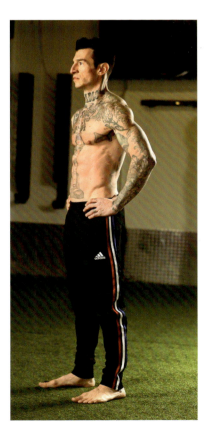
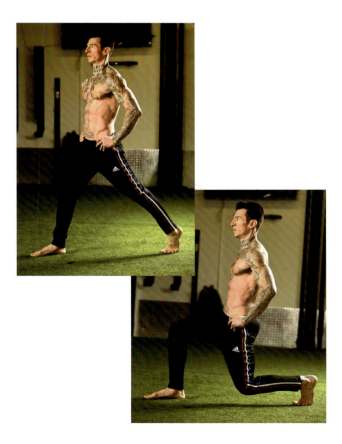

WEIGHTED LUNGE

Adding external resistance to this dynamic exercise requires extra control, so that the momentum of the weight does not take over.

1 - Stand up straight with a dumbbell or kettlebell in each hand and your feet approximately shoulder width apart, then take a big step back with one leg.

2 - Keep your entire front foot on the ground, while allowing your rear heel to come up. Keep your chest up and lower yourself down, bending both knees to approximately 90°. Do not let your rear knee touch the ground.

3 - Drive your front heel and rear toe into the ground to bring your rear leg forward and your feet together again. Alternate sides between repetitions.

Trainer Talk: Lunges can also be done in a walking pattern, where you continually step forward from rep to rep.

Primary Muscles: Quadriceps, hamstrings, glutes.
Secondary Muscles: Calves, tibialis.

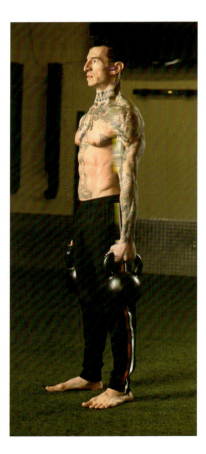
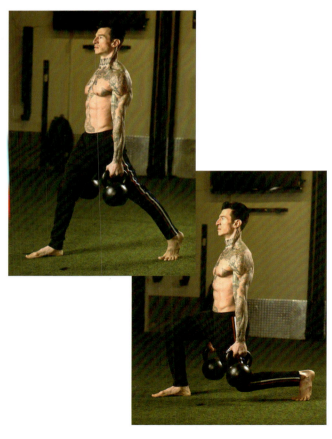

BARBELL LUNGE

Holding the barbell on your back places greater demand on your traps, back and shoulders.

1 - Get under the racked barbell so that it rests on your traps, just above your posterior deltoids. Grasp the bar tightly with your chest up, and your feet approximately shoulder width apart. Step back and remove the bar from the rack. Take a big step back with one leg.

2 - Keep your entire front foot on the ground, while allowing your rear heel to come up. Keep your chest up and lower yourself down, bending both knees to approximately 90°. Do not let your rear knee touch the ground.

3 - Drive your front heel and rear toe into the ground to bring your rear leg forward and your feet together again. Alternate sides between repetitions.

Trainer Talk: Because of the size of a barbell, this lunge variant does not loan itself as well to walking as the others.

Primary Muscles: Quadriceps, hamstrings, glutes.

Secondary Muscles: Calves, tibialis.

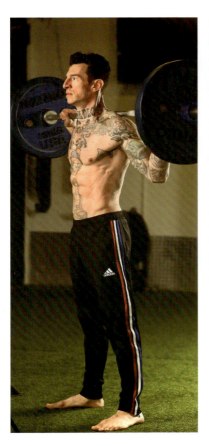
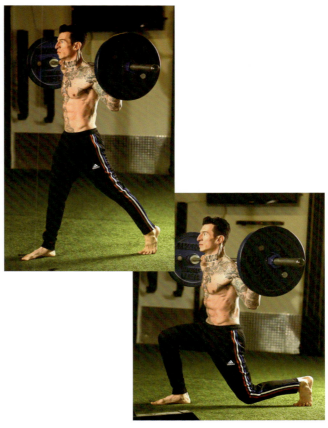

BULGARIAN SPLIT SQUAT

Elevating your rear foot in a Bulgarian split squat places a greater amount of bodyweight into the forward foot than a traditional split squat does.

1 - Stand in front of a bench or step. Lift one foot and place it on the bench or step behind you.

2 - Keep your back straight and chest up as you lower yourself down until your front knee bends to approximately 90°. Your rear knee will be bent to a more acute angle.

3 - Pause briefly at the bottom before returning to the top position, keeping your rear foot on the bench. Complete your set in its entirety and then repeat on the opposite side.

Trainer Talk: Keep your front foot totally flat. Your rear foot can either rest on the ball and toes or on top of the foot.

Primary Muscles: Quadriceps, hamstrings, glutes.

Secondary Muscles: Calves, tibialis.

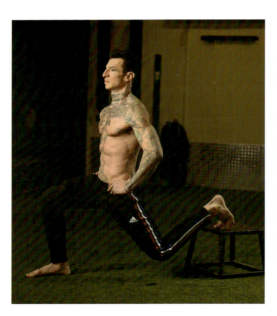
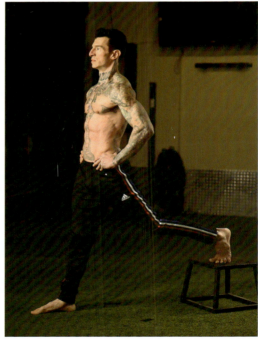

WEIGHTED BULGARIAN SPLIT SQUAT

Adding external resistance to this bodyweight classic is an excellent way to train harder, employ more of your core and trigger greater muscular growth, without having to incorporate a different movement pattern. Dumbbells and kettlebells work better than a barbell due to the mechanics of this exercise.

1 - Stand in front of a bench or step with a dumbbell or kettlebell in each hand. Lift one foot and place it on the bench or step behind you.

2 - Keep your back straight and chest up as you lower yourself down until your front knee bends to approximately 90°. Your rear knee will be bent to a more acute angle.

3 - Pause briefly at the bottom before returning to the top position, keeping your rear foot on the bench. Complete your set in its entirety and then repeat on the opposite side.

Trainer Talk: Keep your front foot totally flat. Your rear foot can either rest on the ball and toes or on top of the foot.

Primary Muscles: Quadriceps, hamstrings, glutes.

Secondary Muscles: Calves, tibialis.

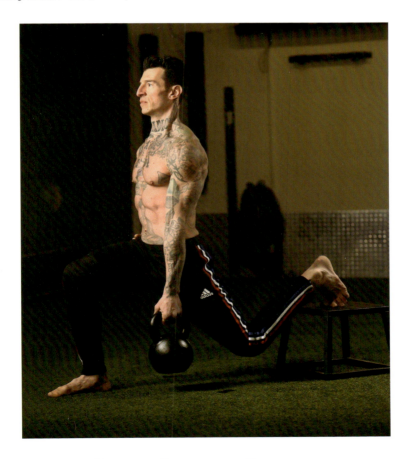

ONE LEG SQUAT

One leg squats are the ultimate fusion of strength, balance and flexibility. Take this exercise slowly, especially in the lowering phase.

1 - Stand on a bench or step with one foot. Allow the non-standing leg to hang off.

2 - Reach your arms forward and squat down with your standing leg, until your hamstrings make contact with your calf. Be sure to keep your foot flat the entire time. Allow your non-squatting leg to drop below the step.

3 - Pause briefly at the bottom before returning to the top position. Complete your set in its entirety and then repeat on the opposite side.

Trainer Talk: By standing on a bench, you allow your non-squatting leg to drop below standing level.

Primary Muscles: Quadriceps, hamstrings, glutes.

Secondary Muscles: Spinal erectors, hip flexors, calves.

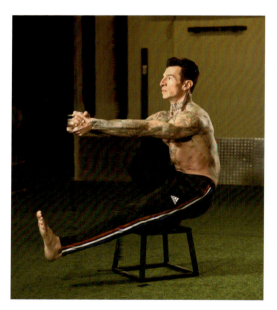 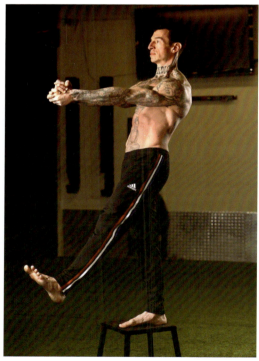

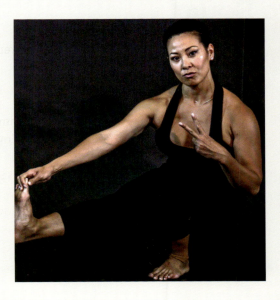

PISTOL SQUAT

A "pistol" squat is a one leg squat variant where you stand directly on the ground rather than on a bench. This position demands greater hamstrings flexibility. Grabbing the toe of your extended foot will help you keep your leg straight and close the kinetic chain of tension in the body.

ASSIST YOURSELF

Self-assistance is a key principle in progressive calisthenics. If you are lacking in strength, balance or mobility, simply getting a feel for the complete range of motion can be very helpful, even if the full expression of an exercise is out of reach. If you're having a hard time with the one leg squat, try grabbing a pole, squat rack or any sturdy object so you can help yourself up if necessary. The idea is to assist yourself as little as possible, so don't pull any more than you need to. In time you will need less and less self-assistance, until you can eliminate it completely.

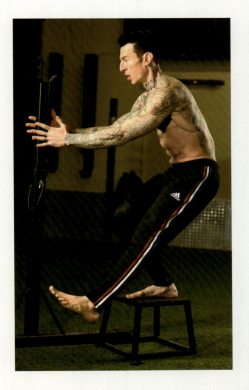

WEIGHTED ONE LEG SQUAT

Adding external resistance to this bodyweight classic is an excellent way to train harder, employ more of your core and trigger greater muscular growth, without having to incorporate a different movement pattern. Dumbbells and kettlebells work well for weighted one leg squats.

1 - Grasp a dumbbell or kettlebell and stand on a bench or step with one foot. Allow the non-standing leg to hang off.

2 - Squeeze tightly and squat down with your standing leg, until your hamstrings make contact with your calf. Be sure to keep your foot flat the entire time. Allow your opposite leg to drop below the step.

3 - Pause briefly at the bottom before returning to the top position. Complete your set in its entirety and then repeat on the opposite side.

Trainer Talk: Maintain tension in the entire body throughout the duration of this exercise, even in the non-squatting leg.

Primary Muscles: Quadriceps, hamstrings, glutes.

Secondary Muscles: Spinal erectors, rhomboids, hip flexors, calves.

CAUTION! Do not attempt this exercise until you are proficient with unweighted one leg squats. Progress slowly.

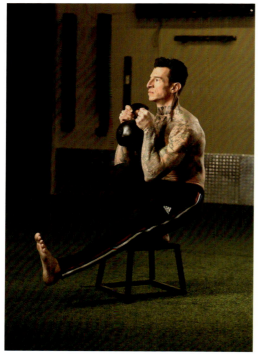
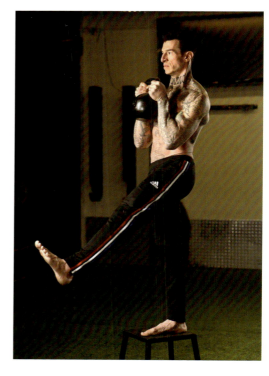

HIP BRIDGE

The hip bridge is helpful for both mobility and strength. Bridging complements squatting and deadlifting very well.

1 - Lie on the ground facing up with your hands by your sides. Keep your knees bent and your feet flat on the floor.

2 - Press your heels into the floor, lifting your hips as high as you can while creating an arch in your back.

3 - Pause briefly before returning to the starting position.

Trainer Talk: Focus on pressing into your heels.

Primary Muscles: Glutes, hamstrings, spinal erectors.

Secondary Muscles: Calves.

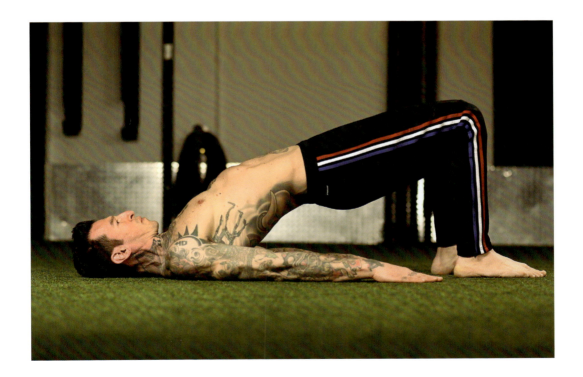

ONE LEG HIP BRIDGE

By performing a hip bridge on one leg, the strength requirement is doubled and a balance element is introduced.

1 - Lie on the ground facing up with your hands by your sides. Keep your knees bent and your feet flat on the floor. Lift one leg straight up and lock at the knee.

2 - Press your grounded heel into the floor, lifting your hips as high as you can while creating an arch in your back.

3 - Pause briefly before returning to the starting position. Complete your set in its entirety and then repeat on the opposite leg.

Trainer Talk: Focus on keeping your hips even.

Primary Muscles: Glutes, hamstrings, spinal erectors.

Secondary Muscles: Calves.

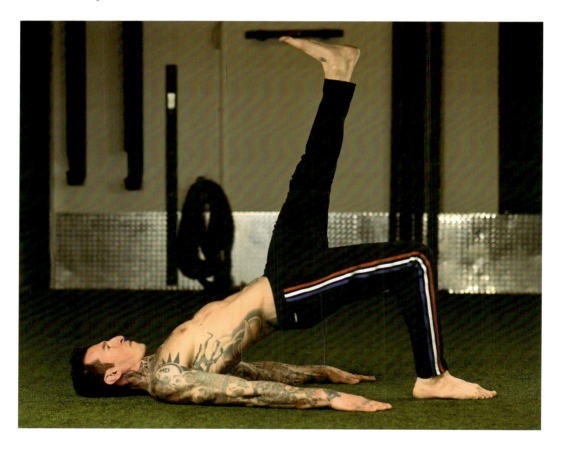

DEADLIFT

The deadlift is one of the three main powerlifting exercises, and also one of the greatest measures of absolute strength. It has a tremendous crossover to real world strength outside the gym.

1 - Stand facing a barbell with your feet approximately shoulder width apart, your chest up and your shoulder blades back. Make sure your shins are close to the bar.

2 - Hinge at your hips and bend your knees, bringing your upper body toward the ground. Grasp the bar and lift by pushing your hips forward, straightening your legs and digging your feet into the floor.

3 - Pause briefly at the top position and then carefully return the bar to the ground being mindful not to flex forward or hyperextend your back.

Trainer Talk: The deadlift uses every muscle in the body. Although it is placed in the "legs" category, it could easily be placed in "back" as well.

Primary Muscles: Hamstrings, glutes, spinal erectors, calves, trapezius, rhomboids, forearms.

Secondary Muscles: All.

CAUTION! Try to avoid any rounding of the back during any deadlift variation. Instead, practice the exercise at a lower weight without compromising form.

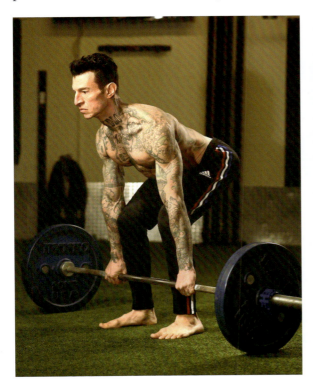 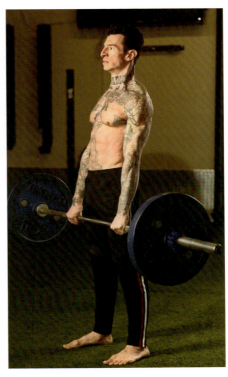

GET A GRIP

When performing a deadlift, the barbell is traditionally grasped using an overhand grip, with your palms facing you. Sometimes a switch grip or lifting straps are employed for assistance. I generally choose not to. My take is, unless you're pulling extremely heavy weight, where you'd need every single advantage you can get, then stick with the traditional grip and get better at it. After all, grip training is part of the exercise.

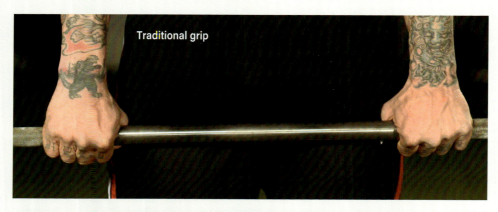

Traditional grip

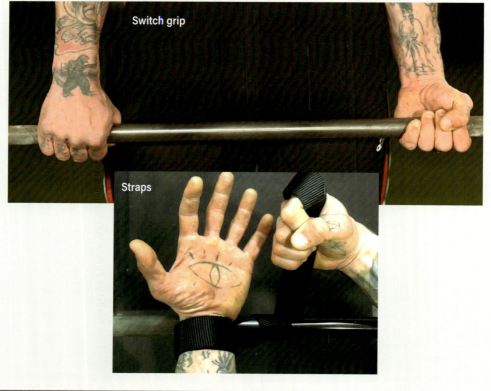

Switch grip

Straps

ROMANIAN DEADLIFT

The Romanian deadlift is a variation where you hinge deeper at the hips and don't bend your knees as much. This places a greater emphasis on the hamstrings, glutes and spinal erectors.

1 - Stand facing a barbell with your feet approximately shoulder width apart, your chest up and your shoulder blades back. Make sure your shins are close to the bar.

2 - Hinge deeply at your hips and bend your knees ever so slightly, bringing your upper body toward the ground. Grasp the bar and lift by pushing your hips forward, straightening your legs and digging your feet into the floor.

3 - Pause briefly at the top position and then carefully return the bar to the ground being mindful not to flex forward or hyperextend your back.

Trainer Talk: Due to deeper hinging of the body, the Roumanian deadlift requires greater hip and hamstring flexibility than the traditional deadlift

Primary Muscles: Hamstrings, glutes, spinal erectors, calves, trapezius, rhomboids, forearms.

Secondary Muscles: All.

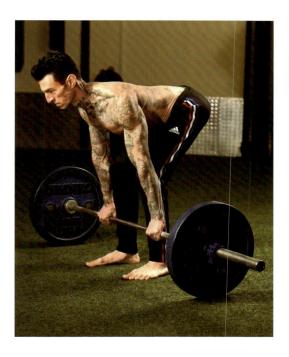
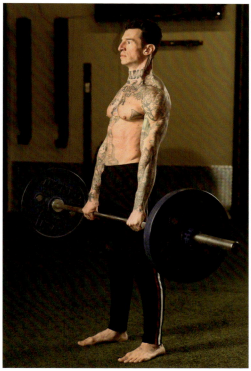

SUMO STANCE

The sumo stance deadlift is a variant in which the practitioner stands with their feet far wider than shoulders and their knees and toes pointed out. The bar is still grasped approximately shoulder width. This position targets the adductors more than a classic deadlift, and places less emphasis on the lower back, as it requires less of a pelvic tilt.

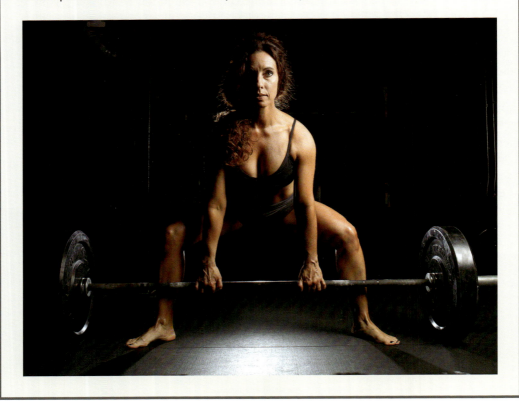

TRAP BAR DEADLIFT

A trap bar is a specialty bar where two parallel bars are welded to a hexagonal frame. Using a trap bar while deadlifting allows you to position your palms facing one another. This is a more structurally sound grip that generally allows for greater overall pull.

1 - Stand centered in a trap bar with your feet approximately shoulder width apart, your chest up and your shoulder blades back.

2 - Hinge at your hips and bend your knees, bringing your upper body toward the ground and grasp the bar, making sure you center your hand on the bars. Your chest will not be as close to the ground as with a traditional deadlift. Grasp and lift the bar by pushing your hips forward, straightening your legs and digging your feet into the floor.

3 - Pause briefly at the top position and then carefully return the bar to the ground being mindful not to flex forward or hyperextend your back.

Trainer Talk: The trap bar places less weight in the lumbar spine than a traditional bar. Since the weight is positioned centrally along the body instead of in front of it, there is less of a forward lean.

Primary Muscles: Hamstrings, glutes, spinal erectors, calves, trapezius, latissimus dorsi, rhomboids.

Secondary Muscles: All.

CAUTION! Make sure you grab each side of the bar in the center, so the total weight is evenly distributed, and the bar does not tilt forward or back.

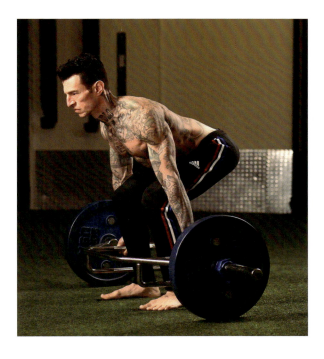
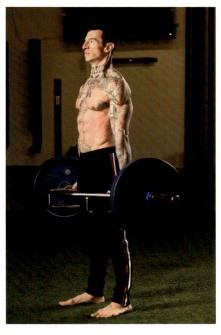

ON CALVES

There are no calf-specific exercises in this book. Some may disagree, but I feel that calf isolation-style exercises are not an effective use of time for most people. We spoke of primary exercises (deadlift or pull-up for example) and secondary exercises (lat raise or dumbbell curl for example.) Calf exercises would be tertiary. When you train squats, lunges, deadlifts and more, you work your calves. Calf isolation-style exercises do exist, but they are not part of this program. Unless you're a competitive bodybuilder, or have a particular reason to isolate calves, then there are simply more efficient ways to work out.

LEG STRETCH #1
QUADRICEPS STRETCH

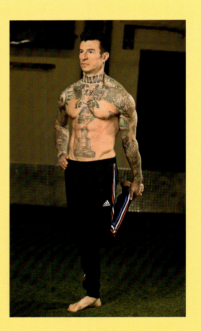

1 - Stand up straight and bend your leg at the knee. Grab it just above the foot.

2 - Use your arm to bend your knee so you feel the stretch in your quadriceps.

3 - Hold this position and repeat on the opposite side.

Works: Quadriceps, hip flexors.

LEG STRETCH #2
HIP FLEXORS STRETCH

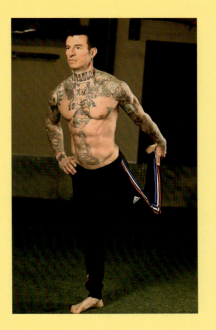

1 - Stand up straight and bend your leg at the knee. Grab it just above the foot.

2 - Use your arm to bend your hip and knee so you feel the stretch in your hip flexors, not just your quadriceps.

3 - Hold this position and repeat on the opposite side.

Works: Hip flexors, quadriceps.

LEG STRETCH #3
HAMSTRINGS STRETCH

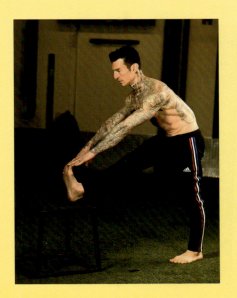

1 - Stand up and place one heel up on a bench. Keep your leg straight and lean forward toward the elevated foot.

2 - Make sure you keep your hips even and level with each other. Lean in as far as you can.

3 - Hold this position and repeat on the opposite side.

Works: Hamstrings, spinal erectors, glutes.

LEG STRETCH #4
FORWARD BEND

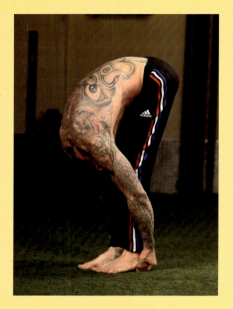

1 - Stand up with your feet together and heels touching. Sweep your arms over your head and interlace your fingers. Release the index finger and reach overhead.

2 - Keep your biceps as close to your ears as you can, bend from your hips and lean forward. Try to get your chest as close to your thighs as possible. Bend your knees if needed.

3 - Grab the back of your heels and pull with your arms as you press your heels into the ground for a deeper stretch. Hold and return to the starting position.

Works: Hamstrings, glutes, calves, spinal erectors, latissimus dorsi, rhomboids.

CHEST

1. Push-up
2. Incline Push-up
3. Decline push-up
4. One Arm Push-up
5. Barbell Bench Press
6. Dumbbell Bench Press
7. Incline Barbell Bench Press
8. Incline Dumbbell Bench Press
9. Dumbbell Fly
10. Incline Dumbbell Fly
11. Dumbbell Pullover
12. Chest Stretches

PUSH-UP

The push-up is the foundational upper body exercise. Push-ups (or incline push-ups) are a prerequisite for any type of bench press.

1 - Place your hands on the ground approximately shoulder width apart. Keep your feet together and form a straight line from your head to your heels.

2 - Bend at the elbows and shoulders and lower your chest toward the floor. Allow your shoulder blades to come together as your chest descends.

3 - Pause briefly with your chest approximately one inch from the ground. Allow your shoulder blades to spread apart as you press yourself back to the starting position.

Trainer Talk: A wider hand position places greater emphasis on the pectorals. A narrower hand position places greater emphasis on the triceps.

Primary Muscles: Pectorals, triceps.

Secondary Muscles: Anterior deltoids, abdominals.

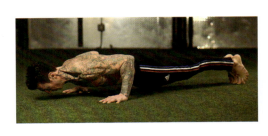

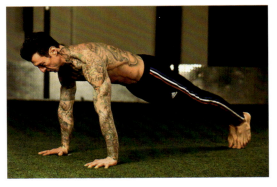

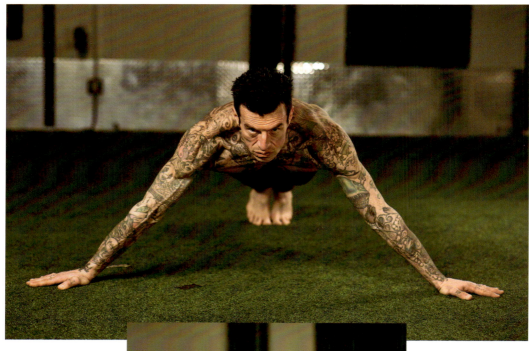

A wider hand position places greater emphasis on the pectoral muscles. A narrower hand position places greater emphasis on the triceps. Just make sure that your elbows track below the shoulders to avoid any shearing.

INCLINE PUSH-UP

Elevating your hands in an incline push-up places less bodyweight into the upper body than a traditional push-up does.

1 - Place your hands on a bench approximately shoulder width apart. Keep your feet together on the ground and form a straight line from your head to your heels.

2 - Bend at the elbows and shoulders and lower your chest toward the bench. Allow your shoulder blades to come together as your chest descends.

3 - Pause briefly with your chest approximately one inch from the bench. Allow your shoulder blades to spread apart as you press yourself back to the starting position.

Trainer Talk: This is an important exercise if you're struggling with push-ups. The higher you place your hands, the more forgiving the exercise becomes. Beginners are encouraged to use a high bench.

Primary Muscles: Pectorals, triceps.
Secondary Muscles: Anterior deltoids, abdominals.

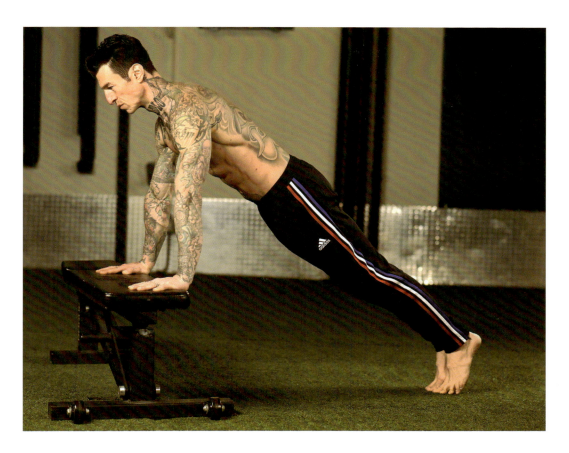

DECLINE PUSH-UP

Elevating your feet in a decline push-up places more bodyweight into the upper body than a traditional push-up does.

1 - With a bench behind you, place your hands on the ground approximately shoulder width apart. Place your feet together on the bench, forming a straight line from your head to your heels.

2 - Bend at the elbows and shoulders and lower your chest toward the floor. Allow your shoulder blades to come together as your chest descends.

3 - Pause briefly with your chest approximately one inch from the ground. Allow your shoulder blades to spread apart as you press yourself back to the starting position.

Trainer Talk: This exercise is the inverse of an incline push-up. The higher you place your feet, the more difficult the exercise becomes.

Primary Muscles: Pectorals, triceps.

Secondary Muscles: Anterior deltoids, abdominals.

CAUTION! Decline push-ups can place a lot of stress on the wrists for some people. If you have wrist issues or are recovering from an injury, be extra careful.

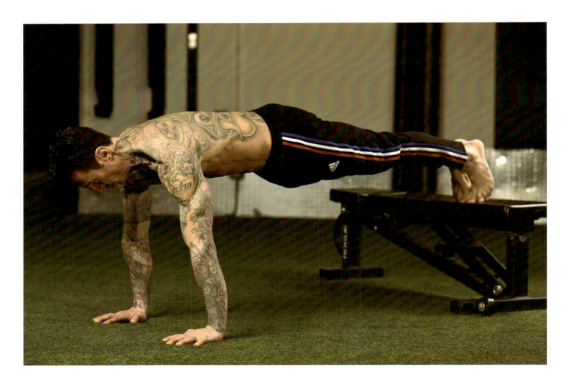

ONE ARM PUSH-UP

The one arm push-up is a classic bodyweight feat of strength. Don't be fooled by the name, as this exercise demands full body tension, as well as a keen neurology.

1 - Place your hands close together on the ground with your feet apart. Engage your entire body and remove one hand from the floor, placing it at your side.

2 - Bend the elbow of your pressing arm and lower your chest toward the floor. Keep your elbow close to your side and your shoulders even.

3 - Pause briefly with your chest approximately one inch from the ground, then press yourself back to the starting position. Try to avoid any bending at all from your hips or low back. Complete your set in its entirety and then repeat on the opposite side.

Trainer Talk: Be careful to maintain tension in your non-pressing arm and keep your shoulders even. The shoulder of the non-pressing arm should not come up sooner than the shoulder of the pressing arm.

Primary Muscles: Pectorals, triceps.

Secondary Muscles: Anterior deltoids, abdominals, glutes.

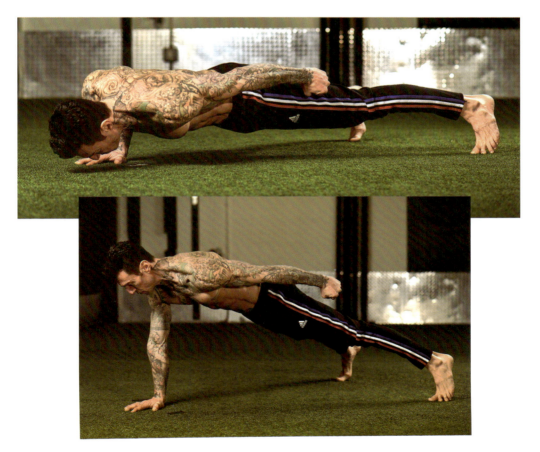

ASSIST YOURSELF

Self-assistance is a key principle in progressive calisthenics. If you are lacking in strength, balance or mobility, simply getting a feel for the full range of motion of an exercise can be very helpful. If you're having a hard time with the one arm push-up, try giving yourself a little help with the non-pressing hand, even just a few fingers. The idea is to assist yourself as little as possible, so don't press any more than you need to. You can also perform this exercise on an incline. As with classic two-arm push-ups, elevating the upper body provides a mechanical advantage. The higher you place your hand, the better the leverage.

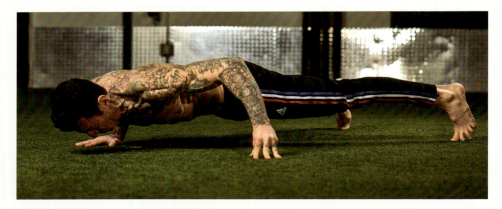

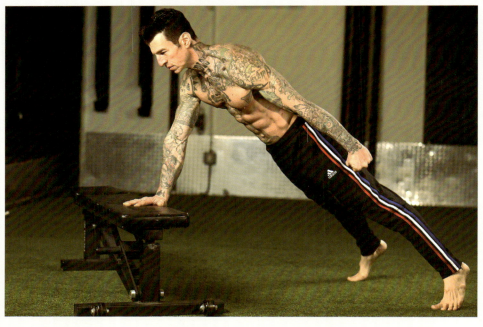

BARBELL BENCH PRESS

The barbell bench press (aka chest press is one of the three main powerlifting exercises. Using a barbell allows you to push the maximum absolute weight as compared to dumbbells or bodyweight (push-ups).

1 - Lie down on a bench with your feet flat on the floor and your body braced. Lift your chest and slightly arch your back. Place your hands on the bar slightly wider than shoulder width so that your forearms are perpendicular to the ground. Unrack the bar and extend your arms.

2 - Bend at the elbows and shoulders and lower the bar toward your chest. Do not bounce the bar off your chest.

3 - Extend your arms to press the bar back to starting position.

Trainer Talk: The push-up (or incline push-up) is a prerequisite to the barbell bench press. As with the push-up, you may experiment with different hand positions. A wider hand position places greater emphasis on the pectorals. A narrower hand position places greater emphasis on the triceps.

Primary Muscles: Pectorals, triceps.

Secondary Muscles: Anterior deltoids.

CAUTION! The combination of lifting heavy weight on a fixed bar and the shallow structure of the shoulder socket can lead to potential shoulder discomfort. As an alternative, you may use dumbbells, as they allow for a more natural movement at the shoulder joint. (See next exercise.) Use a spotter for heavy weight.

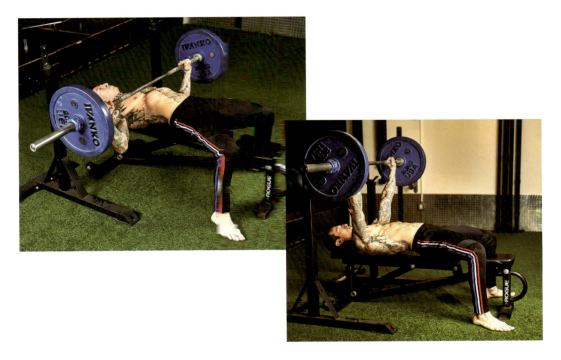

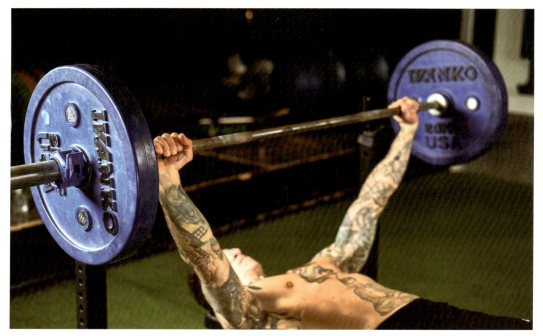

A wider hand position places greater emphasis on the pectorals muscles.

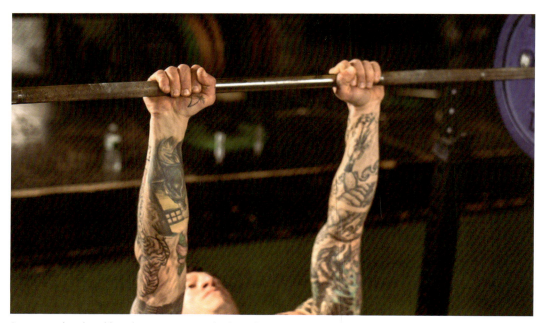

A narrower hand position places greater emphasis on the triceps and deltoids. Just make sure that your elbows track below the shoulders to avoid any shearing.

DUMBBELL BENCH PRESS

When using dumbbells, each arm functions on its own without being fixed to the other. Because of this, you must employ more stabilizer muscles. You can also achieve greater and more natural range of motion.

1 - Lie down on a bench with your feet flat on the floor and your body braced. Lift your chest and slightly arch your back. Hold the dumbbells above your chest with your arms extended.

2 - Bend at the elbows and shoulders and lower the dumbbells toward your chest.

3 - Extend your arms to press the dumbbells back to starting position. You may rotate at the shoulders.

Trainer Talk: The same reasons that allow for a more natural movement pattern than a barbell does will also prohibit you from lifting as heavy as you could with a barbell.

Primary Muscles: Pectorals, triceps.

Secondary Muscles: Anterior deltoids.

CAUTION! Don't let your elbows flare out too wide or high. Keep them beneath your shoulders, somewhat close to your torso.

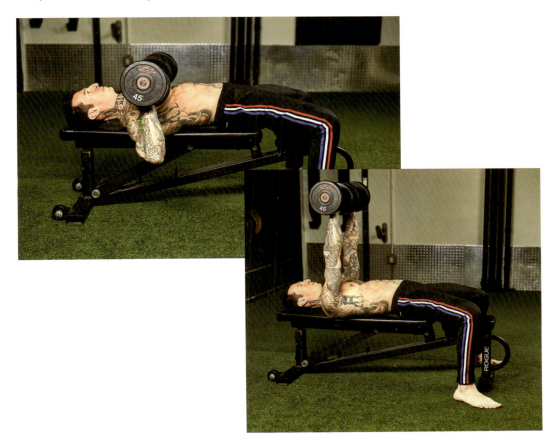

INCLINE BARBELL BENCH PRESS

Performing a bench press on an incline of about 45° - 60° targets the chest from a different angle and emphasizes the upper pectorals muscles.

1 - Sit down on an incline bench with your feet flat on the floor and your body braced. Lift your chest and slightly arch your back. Place your hands on the bar slightly wider than shoulder width so that your forearms are perpendicular to the ground. Unrack the bar and extend your arms.

2 - Bend at the elbows and shoulders and lower the bar toward your chest. Do not bounce the bar off your chest.

3 - Extend your arms to press the bar back to starting position.

Trainer Talk: Even though your body is positioned on an angle, make sure that your forearms still track perpendicular to the ground. Use a spotter for heavy weight.

Primary Muscles: Pectorals, triceps.

Secondary Muscles: Anterior deltoids.

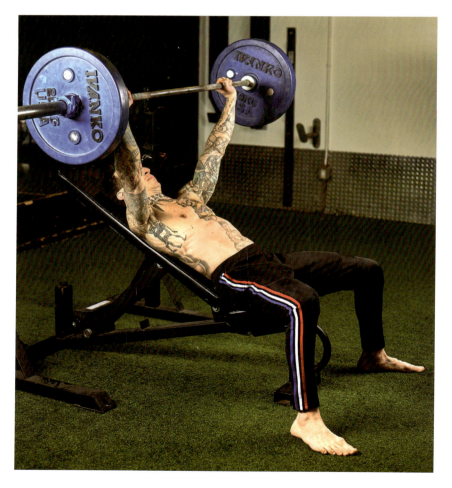

INCLINE DUMBBELL BENCH PRESS

Performing a dumbbell bench press on an incline of about 45° - 60° targets the chest from a different angle and emphasizes the upper pectorals and anterior deltoids more than a flat dumbbell bench press does.

1 - Sit down on an incline bench with your feet flat on the floor and your body braced. Lift your chest and slightly arch your back. Hold the dumbbells above your chest with your arms extended.

2 - Bend at the elbows and shoulders and lower the dumbbells toward your chest.

3 - Extend your arms to press the dumbbells back to starting position. You may rotate at the shoulders.

Trainer Talk: Even though your body is positioned on an angle, make sure that your forearms still track perpendicular to the ground.

Primary Muscles: Pectorals, triceps.

Secondary Muscles: Anterior deltoids.

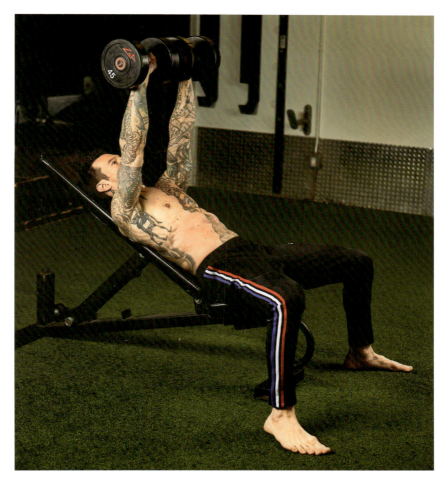

DUMBBELL FLY

It's easy to forget that your pecs don't just push and press. They are also adductors. Flys target your chest in this capacity, and also increase flexibility. The fly is a "light weight" or secondary exercise. It is a spectacular complement to the larger movements that recruit more (or bigger) muscles and yield greater energy expenditure.

1 - Lie down on a bench with your feet flat on the floor and your body braced. Hold the dumbbells facing each other above your chest with your elbows slightly bent to relieve stress on the joints.

2 - Maintain the *slight* bend in your elbows and open your arms until they are approximately parallel to the ground.

3 - Lift the dumbbells from the chest without changing the degree of elbow flexion, and bring the dumbbells together gently over your chest.

Trainer Talk: The movement pattern of the dumbbell fly is often compared to "hugging a tree".

Primary Muscles: Pectorals.

Secondary Muscles: N/A

CAUTION! Do not perform dumbbell flys with heavy weights.

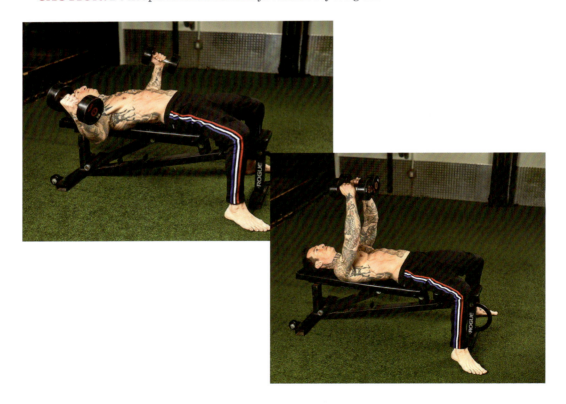

Incline Dumbbell Fly

Performing dumbbell flys on an incline of about 45° - 60° targets the chest from a different angle and emphasizes the upper pectorals more than flat dumbbell flys do.

1 - Sit down on an incline bench with your feet flat on the floor and your body braced. Hold the dumbbells facing each other above your chest with your elbows slightly bent to relieve stress on the joints.

2 - Maintain the slight bend in your elbows and open your arms until they are approximately parallel to the ground.

3 - Lift the dumbbells from the chest without changing the degree of elbow flexion, and bring the dumbbells together gently over your chest.

Trainer Talk: Even though your body is positioned at an angle, make sure that your arms are perpendicular to the ground in the top position.

Primary Muscles: Pectorals.

Secondary Muscles: N/A

CAUTION! Do not perform incline dumbbell flys with heavy weights.

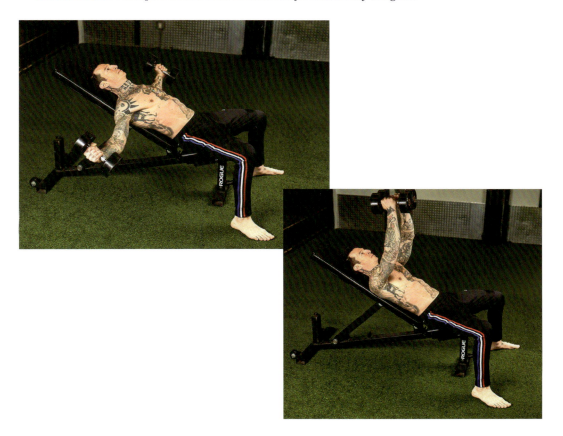

DUMBBELL PULLOVER

The pullover is a unique exercise that is both a push and a pull. It targets the chest as well as the back and also helps with mobility. Although a pullover can also be done with a barbell, I feel the dumbbell provides a more natural feel for the wrists and shoulders.

1 - Lie down on a bench with your feet flat on the floor and your body braced. Lift your chest and slightly arch your back. Hold a dumbbell from the weighted end in both hands, with your thumbs crossed around the handle.

2 - Lower the dumbbell behind your head, descending from your shoulders and bending at your elbows.

3 - Extend your arms to raise the dumbbell back to starting position.

Trainer Talk: The pullover uses many muscles in the upper body. Although it is placed in the "chest" category, it could easily be placed in "back" or "arms" as well.

Primary Muscles: Pectorals, triceps, latissimus dorsi.

Secondary Muscles: Serratus anterior, deltoids, rhomboids.

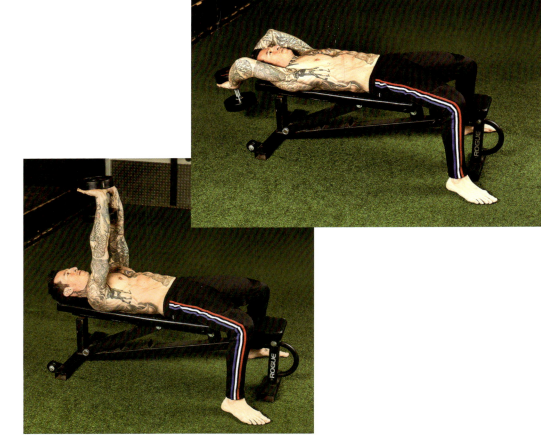

Pullover grip.

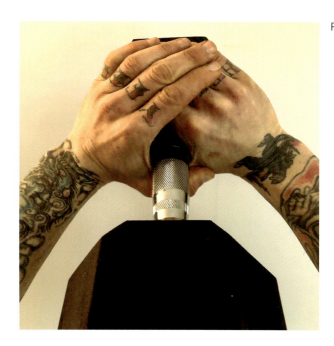

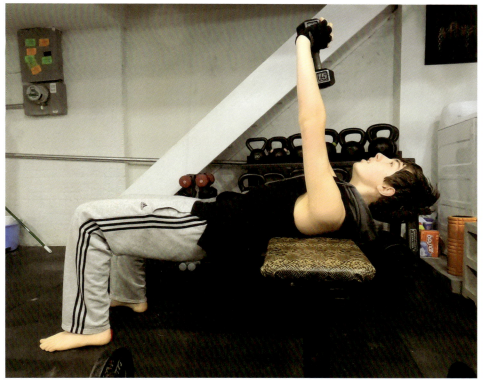

Dumbbell pullovers can also be performed laying perpendicular to the bench. Keep your upper back in contact with the bench, with your hips off the bench and closer to the ground than your upper body.

CHEST STRETCH #1
POLE ASSISTED

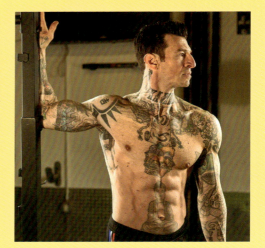

1 - Stand up and place your arm straight out, bent to 90° at the elbow so that your forearm is perpendicular to the ground.

2 - Place your forearm against a pole or wall, pressing it against the surface and rotate your body away. Use the pole for leverage.

3 - Hold this position and repeat on the opposite side.

Works: Pectorals, anterior deltoids, biceps.

CHEST STRETCH #2
HANDS BEHIND BACK

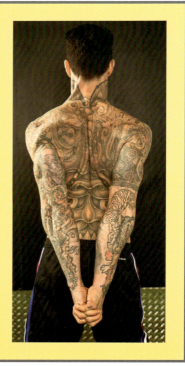

1 - Stand up tall, lift your chest and bring your hands behind your back, interlacing your fingers.

2 - Press the heels of your hands together and keep your arms straight (or as straight as you can).

3 - Bring your shoulder blades together and actively bring your arms closer together behind you so that your biceps go behind your back.

Works: Pectorals, anterior deltoids, abdominals.

BACK

1. Bodyweight Row
2. Barbell Row
3. One Arm Dumbbell Row
4. V Pull-up
5. Pull-up

6. Chin-up
7. Weighted Pull-up/Chin-up
8. Muscle-up
9. Back Stretches

BODYWEIGHT ROW

The bodyweight row (aka Australian pull-up or plank pull) is an upper body pulling exercise. The movement pattern is almost the opposite of a push-up, in that you pull in a horizontal plane instead of push.

1 - Grasp a bar of approximately waist height. Get under the bar and extend your legs in front of you, with your knees bent and feet flat on the ground. Keep your entire body engaged and do not bend your hips.

2 - Bend at the elbows and shoulders and pull your chest toward the bar.

3 - Pause briefly when your chest almost touches the bar, then lower yourself back to the starting position.

Trainer Talk: The bodyweight row can also be performed with your legs straight. Doing so increases the difficulty of the exercise, as it places more of your bodyweight into your upper body.

Primary Muscles: Latissimus dorsi, posterior deltoids, rhomboids.

Secondary Muscles: Biceps, brachialis.

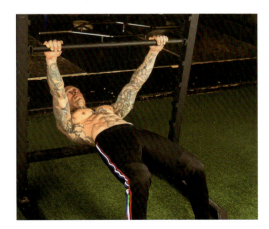 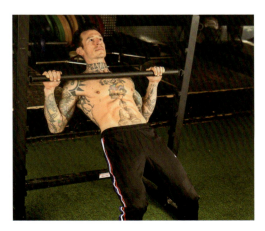

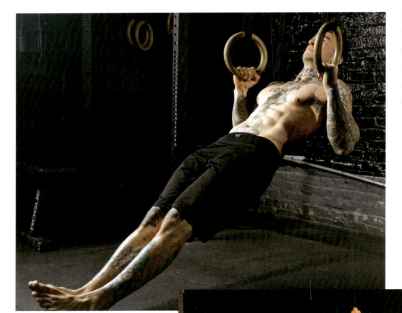

Here is a straight leg bodyweight row performed on gymnastics rings. Rings and suspension trainers are good substitutes if a low bar is not available.

Like a push-up, a bodyweight row can be performed with one arm. When doing so, it is important to maintain tension in the abs, glutes and non-pulling arm.

BARBELL ROW

Unlike bodyweight rows, which involve pulling yourself toward a bar, the barbell row involves pulling the bar to you.

1 - Stand facing a barbell with your feet approximately shoulder width apart, your chest up and your shoulder blades back. Grasp the bar slightly wider than shoulder width with an overhand grip. Bend your hips to approximately 45° and your knees slightly, so that your torso is almost parallel to the ground. Maintain a slight arch in your back.

2 - Keep your body tense and pull the bar toward your chest.

3 - Pause briefly when the bar almost touches your chest, then lower the bar down with control.

Trainer Talk: The barbell row can also be performed with an underhand grip. Doing so places greater emphasis on the biceps and trapezius, and slightly less emphasis on the rhomboids.

Primary Muscles: Latissimus dorsi, posterior deltoids, rhomboids.

Secondary Muscles: Biceps, brachialis, trapezius.

CAUTION! Do not let your back round for any reason. Keep your shoulder blades down and back.

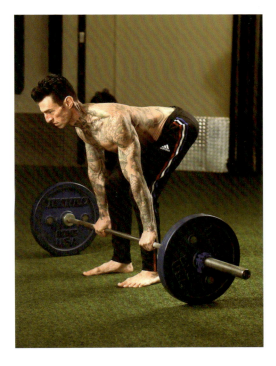
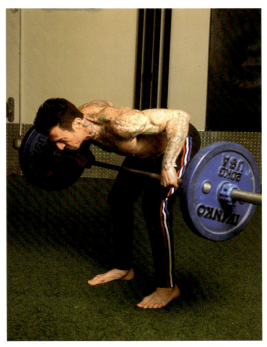

ONE ARM DUMBBELL ROW

Dumbbell rows target the lats one side at a time. The hands are positioned closer together than they are in a barbell row.

1 - Place your hand on a bench with your feet about shoulder width apart, your chest approximately parallel to the ground and your shoulder blades down and back. Grasp a dumbbell with your other hand.

2 - Keep your body tense and pull the dumbbell as high as possible while keeping your shoulders even.

3 - Pause briefly at the top, then lower the dumbbell down with control. Complete your set in its entirety and then repeat on the opposite side.

Trainer Talk: The dumbbell row can also be performed both arms at the same time, without using a bench for support. As with the barbell row, avoid any rounding at the back.

Primary Muscles: Latissimus dorsi, posterior deltoids, rhomboids.

Secondary Muscles: Biceps, brachialis, trapezius.

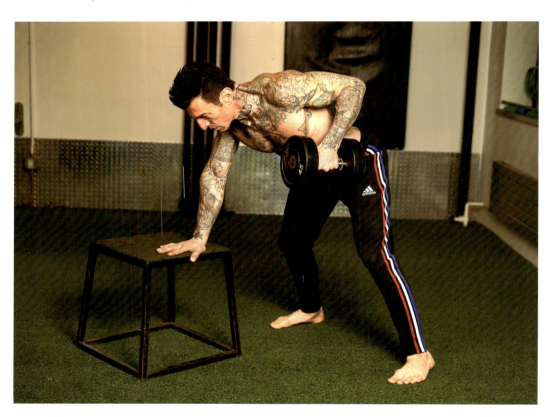

V Pull-up

The V pull-up (aka jackknife pullup) is an excellent progression toward pull-ups, as it mimes the movement pattern, without using all your body weight for resistance.

1 - Grasp an overhead bar in an active hang (see sidebar on page 76) with your palms facing away from you. Bend your hips and place your feet on a step in front of you. Keep your shoulder blades down and back.

2 - Pull yourself up until your chin clears the bar. Avoid shrugging your shoulders or using any momentum.

3 - Lower yourself back to the starting position.

Trainer Talk: Focus on driving your elbows toward your hips in order to fully engage your lats.

Primary Muscles: Latissimus dorsi, rhomboids.

Secondary Muscles: Biceps, brachialis, serratus anterior.

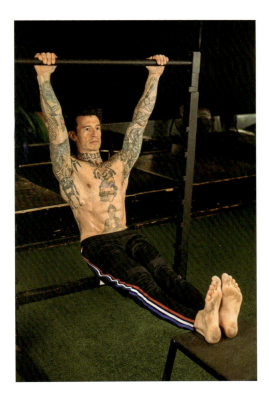

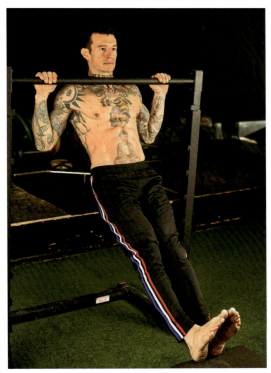

HOW TO HANG

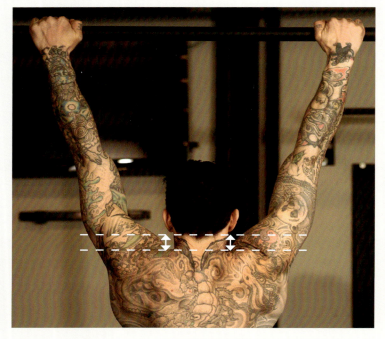

This is a passive hang. Notice how the shoulders are shrugged up by the ears. While this is a great stretch for the lats, spine and shoulders, it is not ideal for initiating pull-ups.

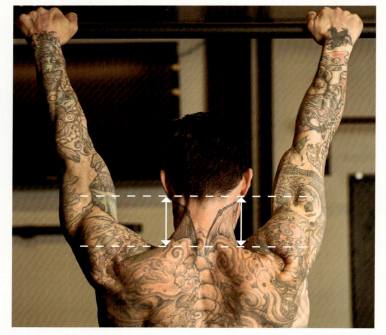

This is an active hang. Notice the space between the ears and shoulders. The muscles in the upper back and abs are engaged. This position is essential before bending your elbows for a pull-up.

PULL-UP

The pull-up is the king of upper body pulling exercises. It is one of the finest measures of relative strength.

1 - Grasp an overhead bar in an active hang (see sidebar on page 76) with your palms facing away from you.

2 - Pull yourself up until your chin clears the bar, keeping your legs straight the whole time. Avoid shrugging your shoulders or using any momentum.

3 - Lower yourself back to the starting position.

Trainer Talk: Focus on driving your elbows toward your hips in order to fully engage your lats. Although the focus is on your upper back and biceps, every muscle in your body should be flexed to get the most out of this exercise.

Primary Muscles: Latissimus dorsi, biceps, brachialis.

Secondary Muscles: Rhomboids, serratus anterior, forearms.

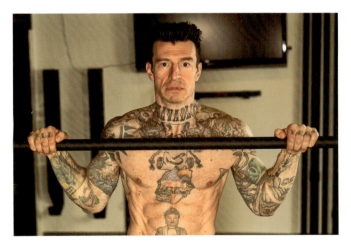

Overhand pull-ups are usually performed with a wide grip for maximum lat activation...

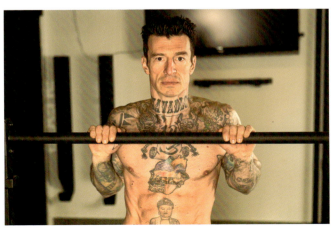

...but they can be performed with a narrow grip as well. Doing so places greater demand on the biceps and forearms.

CHIN-UP

The term "chin-up" is almost interchangeable with "pull-up", except that a chin-up employs an underhand grip, while a pull-up uses an overhand grip.

1 - Grasp an overhead bar in an active hang (see sidebar on page 76) with your palms facing toward you.

2 - Pull yourself up until your chin clears the bar, keeping your legs straight the whole time. Avoid shrugging your shoulders or using any momentum.

3 - Lower yourself back to the starting position.

Trainer Talk: Focus on driving your elbows toward your hips in order to fully engage your lats. Although the focus is on your upper back and biceps, every muscle in your body should be flexed to get the most out of this exercise.

Primary Muscles: Latissimus dorsi, biceps, brachialis.

Secondary Muscles: Rhomboids, serratus anterior, forearms.

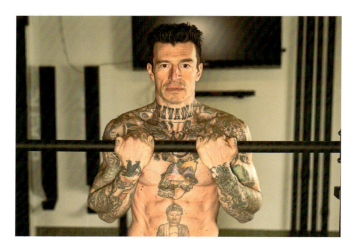

Underhand chin-ups are usually performed with a narrow grip for maximum biceps activation...

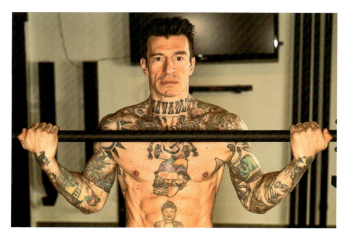

...but they can be performed with a wide grip as well. Doing so places greater demand on the upper back and forearms.

ALTERNATIVE GRIPS

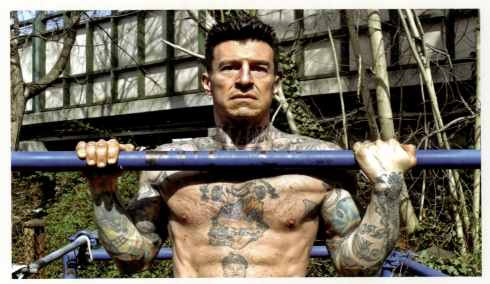

The mixed or "switch" grip is an excellent way to transition from underhand chin-ups to overhand pull-ups. Be mindful to switch which palm is facing you from set to set in order to train each side evenly.

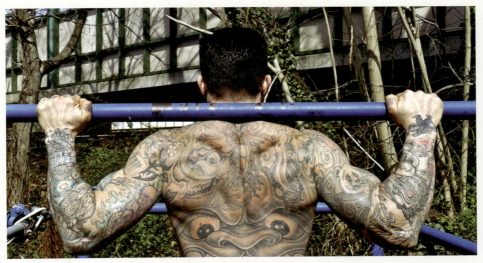

The behind-the-neck pull-up is an advanced variation that recruits the trapezius and rhomboids to a greater degree and improves shoulder mobility. It's important to be comfortable with classic pull-ups before attempting behind-the-neck pull-ups.

PROGRESSING TO PULL-UPS

Let's face it. Pull-ups are hard! If you are having difficulty with pull-ups, you're not alone. Thankfully, there are several different ways to progress.

One approach is to practice your pull-ups with some sort of assistance. Resistance bands are popular because they are inexpensive, portable and available in a variety of resistances. While they have their limitations (such as uneven assistance, mild awkwardness and occasional snappage), bands can be helpful if there is no one else around.

In the case that you have a trainer or partner available, then manual assistance is ideal, as your trainer can control exactly how much (or how little) assistance you'll receive. Plus you won't have to climb into a band.

The lat pulldown is a device that mimics the upper body pulling motion of a pull-up, using a cable and weights. It's typically big and bulky, so I made my own. (It just took a few bucks and a little elbow grease.) Lat pull-downs let you keep your feet on the ground, and allow you to easily change the resistance. To be clear, a lat pull-down is not a pull-up—neither is the bodyweight row for that matter—but they can both help you get there!

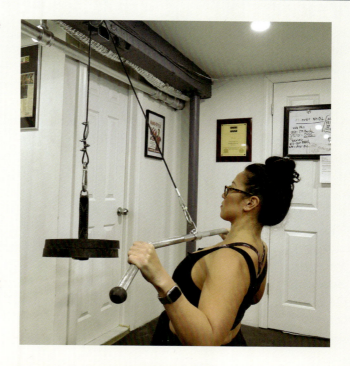

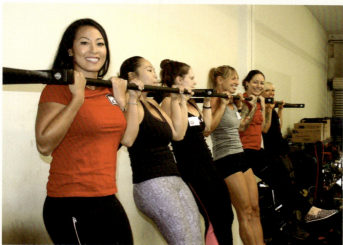

Women generally have more difficulty with pull-ups than men do, due to a lower center of gravity and typically less muscle mass. However, with hard work and consistently—plus these techniques—women can smash pull-ups! We all can!

WEIGHTED PULL-UP/CHIN-UP

Adding external resistance to this bodyweight classic is an excellent way to train harder, employ more of your core and trigger greater muscular growth, without having to incorporate a different movement pattern. A weighted belt, vest or chain work well for weighted pull-ups.

1 - Affix the weight to your body so that it is evenly distributed and does not swing. Grasp an overhead bar in an active hang (see sidebar on page 76) with your palms facing either away from or towards you.

2 - Pull yourself up until your chin clears the bar, keeping your legs straight the whole time. Avoid shrugging your shoulders or using any momentum.

3 - Lower yourself back to the starting position.

Trainer Talk: Weighted pull-ups can potentially place a lot of stress on the elbows. If you have elbow issues or are recovering from an injury, it may be best to avoid weighted pull-ups.

Primary Muscles: Latissimus dorsi, biceps, brachialis.

Secondary Muscles: Rhomboids, serratus anterior, forearms.

CAUTION! Do not attempt this exercise until you are proficient with unweighted pull-ups. Progress slowly.

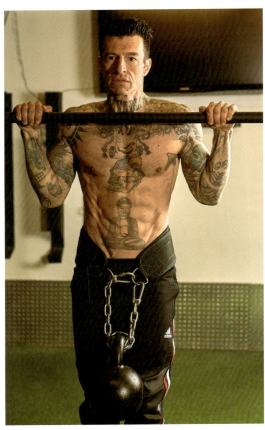

MUSCLE-UP

A muscle-up is a full upper body calisthenics exercise. It's both a push and a pull, as well as a fusion of raw strength and refined technique. The muscle-up is a striking visual that has inspired many to pursue advanced calisthenics.

1 - Grasp an overhead bar in an active hang (see sidebar on page 76) with your palms facing away from you. Position your hands closer together than you would for a standard pull-up.

2 - Pull the bar as low down on your body as possible, using as much force as you can. Bring your elbows above your wrists to help pitch your chest over the bar. Extend your arms to press yourself up, while pushing the bar down.

3 - Lower yourself back to the starting position.

Trainer Talk: The muscle-up defies classification. It is placed in the "back" category because it is an advanced variation of a pull-up. However, it is very much a *full upper body* exercise.

Primary Muscles: Latissimus dorsi, biceps, triceps, pectorals.

Secondary Muscles: Deltoids, rhomboids, serratus anterior, forearms.

CAUTION! Muscle-ups can potentially place a strain on deconditioned shoulders. Make sure you are proficient with pull-ups before attempting.

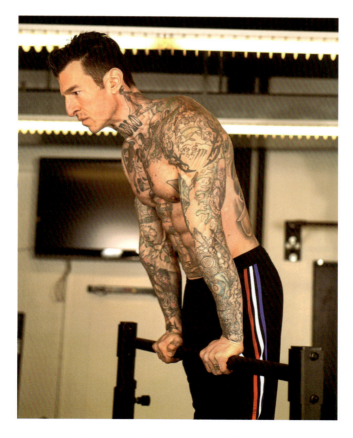

LEADING UP TO MUSCLING UP!

The muscle-up is clearly an advanced exercise, particularly the transition from under the bar to over. Practicing single bar dips (aka straight bar dips) will help you learn this transition over and around the bar. (See page 111 for more info on single bar dips.) Explosive pull-ups are also

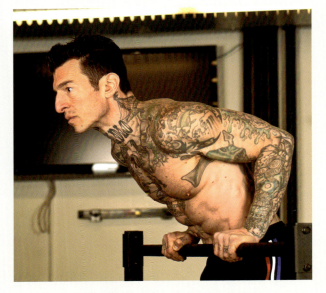

helpful. Pull fast and hard, with your hands (including your thumbs) hooked over the bar to get up as high as possible. Single bar dips and explosive pull-ups are both useful lead up steps to the muscle-up as well as excellent stand-alone exercises.

Single bar dip. Hands are relatively close together.

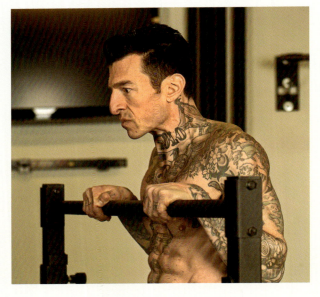

Explosive pull-up. Notice the hook grip.

BACK STRETCH #1
BAR HANG

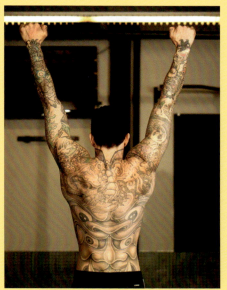

1 - Grasp an overhead bar in a passive hang (see sidebar on page 76) with your palms facing away from you.

2 - Allow your latissimus dorsi to stretch and your vertebrae to separate as your spine lengthens.

3 - Breathe into your spine to lengthen it as you inhale. Allow your lats to extend and your shoulders to shrug as you exhale.

Works: Latissimus dorsi, spine erectors, abdominals, biceps, triceps, forearms, deltoids, trapezius.

BACK STRETCH #2
CRESCENT MOON

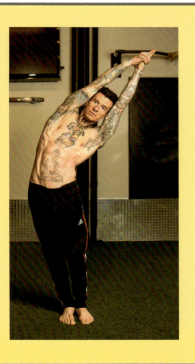

1 - Stand upright and reach your arms overhead, lengthening your body as much as possible.

2 - Press the heels of your hands together and keep your arms straight (or as straight as you can). Keep your biceps pressed against your ears and your chest up.

3 - Lean to the side, pressing your hands up and away, while pushing your hips in the opposite direction. Hold, then go directly to the opposite side, lengthening your body when you pass the center.

Works: Latissimus dorsi, spinal erectors, abdominals, triceps.

BACK STRETCH #3
LOW SQUAT SEMI-HANG

1 - Grasp a bar of approximately waist height with an overhand grip and your arms crossed.

2 - Lower yourself into a deep squat allowing your back to lengthen. Shift your weight from heel to toe, front to back and side to side.

3 - Switch which hand is crossed over on top, to facilitate stretching evenly on both sides.

Works: Latissimus dorsi, rhomboids, posterior deltoids, spinal erectors, glutes.

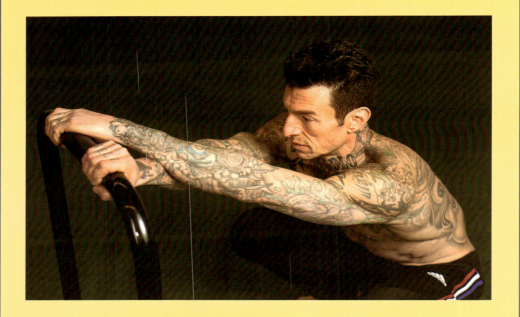

SHOULDERS

1. Standing Overhead Barbell Press
2. Seated Overhead Barbell Press
3. Standing Overhead Dumbbell Press
4. Seated Overhead Dumbbell Press
5. Arnold Press
6. Handstand
7. Handstand Push-up
8. Lateral Raise
9. Front Raise
10. Rear Deltoid Fly
11. Carry
12. Trap Bar Carry
13. Shoulder Stretches

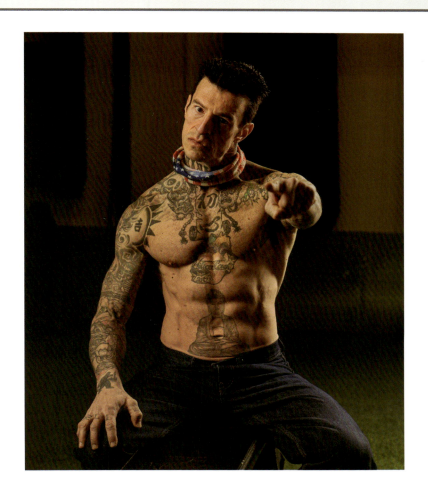

STANDING OVERHEAD BARBELL PRESS

The standing barbell press (aka military press or shoulder press) is the classic shoulder lift.

1 - Stand up straight with your feet flat on the floor and your body braced. Hold a barbell approximately shoulder width across your upper chest using an overhand grip.

2 - Extend at the elbows and shoulders and lift the bar all the way over your head.

3 - Pause briefly before lowering the bar back to the starting position.

Trainer Talk: Try to keep your back straight and avoid excessive arching of the spine.

Primary Muscles: Anterior and medial deltoids, triceps.

Secondary Muscles: Trapezius, pectorals, abdominals.

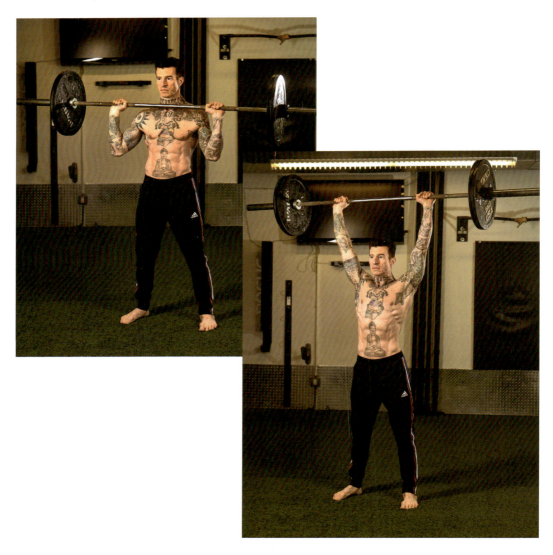

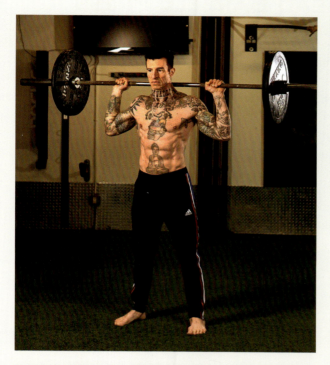

Overhead barbell presses can also be performed lowering the bar behind the neck. This is sometimes referred to as a "back press". This exercise targets the medial and posterior deltoids and helps with shoulder mobility. To avoid injury, take it slow and be careful how low you bring the bar. A back press can be performed standing or seated.

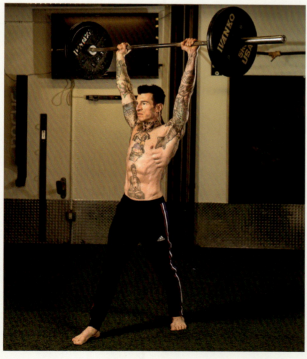

Using a split stance can help eliminate excessive back arching. It gives the lifter a larger footprint for greater support.

SEATED OVERHEAD BARBELL PRESS

By performing this lift from a seated position, pressure is taken off the lower back. Sitting also provides more stability and requires less core recruitment.

1 - Sit up straight on a bench with your feet flat on the floor, your upper back pressed against the backrest and your body braced. Hold a barbell approximately shoulder width across your upper chest using an overhand grip.

2 - Extend at the elbows and shoulders and lift the bar all the way over your head.

3 - Pause briefly before lowering the bar back to the starting position.

Trainer Talk: Try to keep your back straight and avoid arching too much at the spine.

Primary Muscles: Anterior and medial deltoids, triceps.

Secondary Muscles: Trapezius, pectorals.

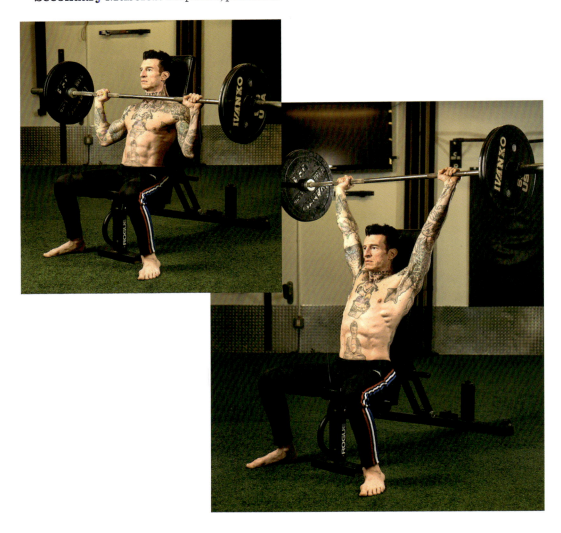

STANDING OVERHEAD DUMBBELL PRESS

When using dumbbells, each arm functions on its own without being fixed to the other. Because of this, you have to maintain stability on your own. You can also achieve a greater and more natural range of motion.

1 - Stand up straight with your feet flat on the floor and your body braced. Hold a pair of dumbbells at your shoulders using an overhand grip.

2 - Extend at the elbows and shoulders and lift the dumbbells all the way over your head.

3 - Pause briefly before lowering the dumbbells back down to the starting position.

Trainer Talk: Try to keep your back straight and avoid arching too much at the spine.

Primary Muscles: Anterior and medial deltoids, triceps.

Secondary Muscles: Trapezius, pectorals, abdominals.

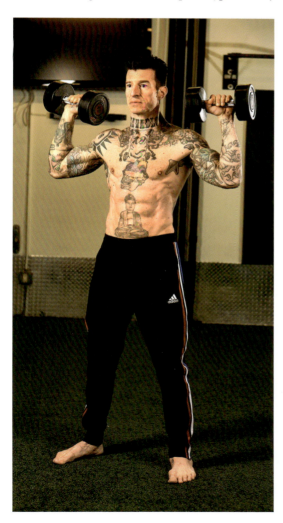
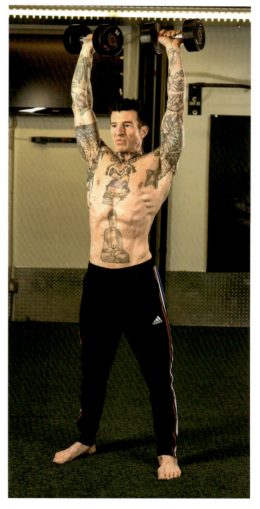

SEATED OVERHEAD DUMBBELL PRESS

By performing this lift from a seated position, pressure is taken off the lower back. Because sitting provides more stability, this variant requires less core recruitment.

1 - Sit up straight on a bench with your feet flat on the floor, your upper back pressed against the backrest and your body braced. Hold a pair of dumbbells at your shoulders using an overhand grip.

2 - Extend at the elbows and shoulders and lift the dumbbells all the way over your head.

3 - Pause briefly before lowering the dumbbells back down to the starting position.

Trainer Talk: Try to keep your back straight and avoid arching too much at the spine.

Primary Muscles: Anterior and medial deltoids, triceps.

Secondary Muscles: Trapezius, pectorals.

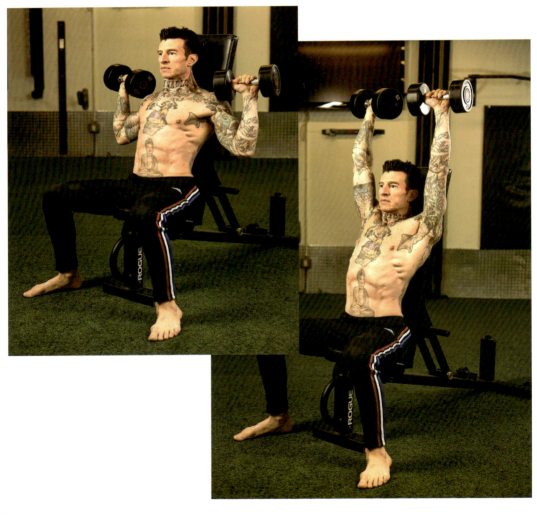

ARNOLD PRESS

Named after the legend himself, this lift is a seated dumbbell press that incorporates shoulder rotation. The Arnold press is excellent for strength building as well as joint mobility.

1 - Sit up straight on a bench with your feet flat on the floor, and your upper back pressed against the backrest. Hold a pair of dumbbells in front of you at shoulder level with an underhand grip and your palms facing toward you.

2 - Extend at the elbows and shoulders, while rotating out at the shoulder and lift the dumbbells all the way over your head. Your grip will switch from underhand to overhand.

3 - Pause briefly before lowering the dumbbells back down to the starting position.

Trainer Talk: Try to keep your back straight and avoid arching too much at the spine.

Primary Muscles: Anterior and medial deltoids, triceps.

Secondary Muscles: Trapezius, pectorals.

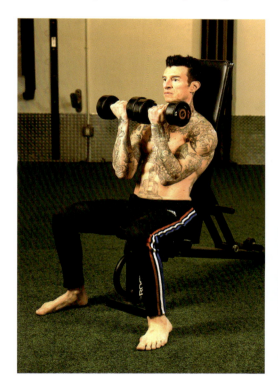

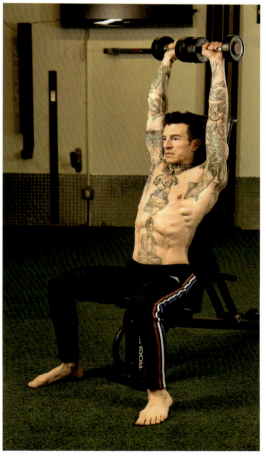

Handstand

This is a wall handstand not a freestanding handstand. The goal here is to focus primarily on strength and complete muscular harmony in the body, while removing some of the balance component.

1 - Place your hands on the floor approximately 6-10 inches away from a wall.

2 - Lock your elbows, brace yourself and kick your legs into the air until your heels come to rest against the wall and press into the ground. Try to feel the entirety of your hand against the floor for maximum stability. Avoid arching too much at the spine.

3 - Hold this position, then come down one leg at a time, as softly as possible.

Trainer Talk: You can also try this facing the wall by starting with your feet and the wall and "walking" yourself up.

Primary Muscles: Deltoids, trapezius.

Secondary Muscles: Pectorals, triceps, abdominals, glutes, forearms.

CAUTION! Handstands can be very spatially confusing. It is a good idea to practice on a padded surface or with a partner.

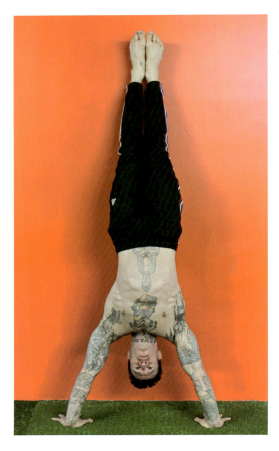

HANDSTAND PUSH-UP

1 - Kick into a handstand against a wall. (See page 94)

2 - Look in between your hands, bend your elbows and shoulders and slowly lower your head toward the ground.

3 - Pause briefly when your face almost touches the floor, then press yourself back to the top, maintaining tension in your entire body.

Trainer Talk: You also try this facing the wall by starting with your feet and the wall and "walking" yourself up.

Primary Muscles: Deltoids, trapezius.

Secondary Muscles: Pectorals, triceps, abdominals, glutes, forearms.

CAUTION! Do not attempt this exercise until you are proficient with wall handstands.

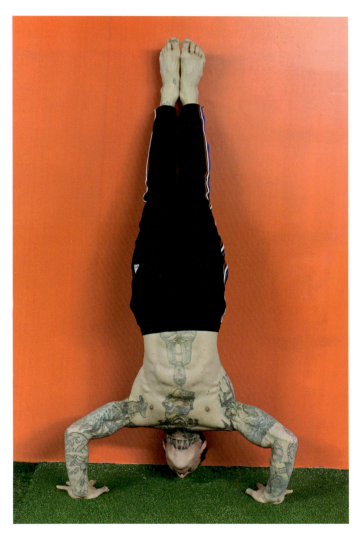

LATERAL RAISE

The lateral raise is a "light weight" or secondary exercise. It is an excellent complement to the larger movements that recruit more (or bigger) muscles and yield greater energy expenditure.

1 - Stand up straight with your feet flat on the floor and your body braced. Hold a pair of dumbbells at your sides.

2 - Maintain a slight bend at your elbows and raise your arms out to your sides until they are parallel to the ground.

3 - Pause briefly before lowering the dumbbells back to the starting position.

Trainer Talk: Lateral raises can be performed standing or seated on a bench. Standing calls for more core recruitment, as the bench provides greater stability.

Primary Muscles: Medial deltoids.

Secondary Muscles: Trapezius.

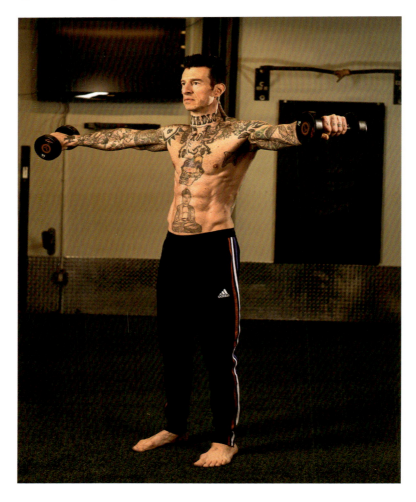

FRONT RAISE

The front raise is a "light weight" or secondary exercise. It is an excellent complement to the larger movements that recruit more (or bigger) muscles and yield greater energy expenditure.

1 - Stand up straight with your feet flat on the floor and your body braced. Hold a pair of dumbbells at your sides using a neutral grip.

2 - Maintain a slight bend at your elbows and raise your arms in front of you until they are parallel to the ground.

3 - Pause briefly before lowering the dumbbells back to the starting position.

Trainer Talk: Front raises can be performed standing or seated on a bench. Standing calls for more core recruitment, as the bench provides greater stability.

Primary Muscles: Anterior deltoids.

Secondary Muscles: Trapezius.

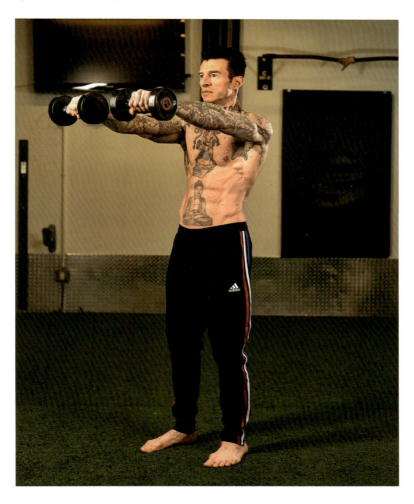

REAR DELTOID FLY

The rear deltoid fly is a "light weight" or secondary exercise. It is an excellent complement to the larger movements that recruit more (or bigger) muscles and yield greater energy expenditure.

1 - Stand up straight with your feet flat on the floor, your knees slightly bent and your body braced. Hold a pair of dumbbells at your sides. Bend your hips to approximately 45° so that your torso is almost parallel to the ground; maintain a slight arch in your back.

2 - Maintain a slight bend at your elbows and raise your arms to your sides until they are parallel to the ground. From this position, this movement targets the rear shoulders.

3 - Pause briefly before lowering the dumbbells back to the starting position.

Trainer Talk: Rear deltoid flys can be performed standing or seated on an incline bench (facedown toward the bench). Standing calls for more core recruitment, as the incline bench provides greater stability.

Primary Muscles: Posterior deltoids.

Secondary Muscles: Trapezius, spinal erectors, rhomboids.

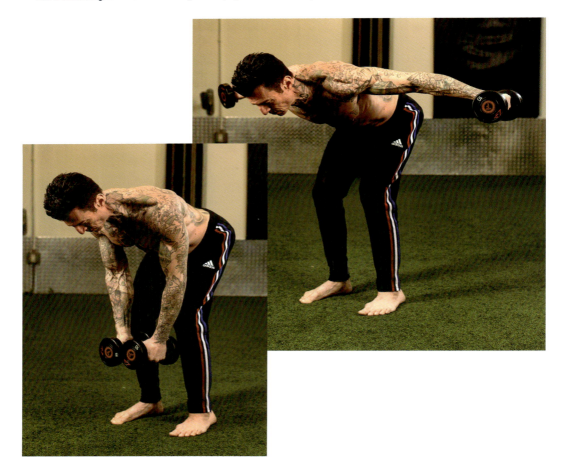

CARRY

The ability to carry heavy weight is, in and of itself, a supreme indicator of strength. The carry (aka farmer's walk) is a classic.

1 - Stand up straight with your feet flat on the floor and your body braced. Hold a dumbbell or kettlebell in each hand. Keep your chest up and shoulder blades back with your hands at your sides.

2 - With your chin level, walk while carrying the weights. Do not let your chin drop.

3 - Set the weights down without letting your shoulders roll forward.

Trainer Talk: Engage your abs and glutes for stability. Avoid excessive arching of the spine.

Primary Muscles: Trapezius, abdominals, pectorals, latissimus dorsi.

Secondary Muscles: Forearms.

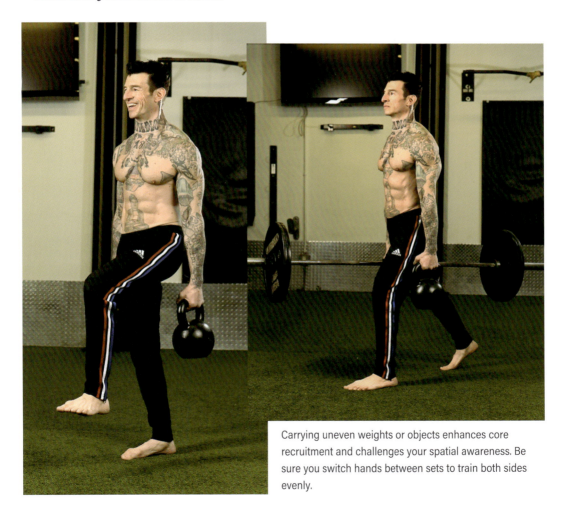

Carrying uneven weights or objects enhances core recruitment and challenges your spatial awareness. Be sure you switch hands between sets to train both sides evenly.

TRAP BAR CARRY

Using a trap bar for carries usually allows for a heavier total load because the sides are fused together and hands stay in a fixed position.

1 - Stand up straight with your feet flat on the floor and your body braced, holding a trap bar. Keep your chest up and your shoulder blades back.

2 - With your chin level, walk while carrying the bar. Do not let your chin drop.

3 - Set the bar down without letting your shoulders roll forward.

Trainer Talk: Make sure you grab each side of the trap bar in the center, so the total weight is evenly distributed.

Primary Muscles: Trapezius, abdominals, pectorals, latissimus dorsi.

Secondary Muscles: Forearms.

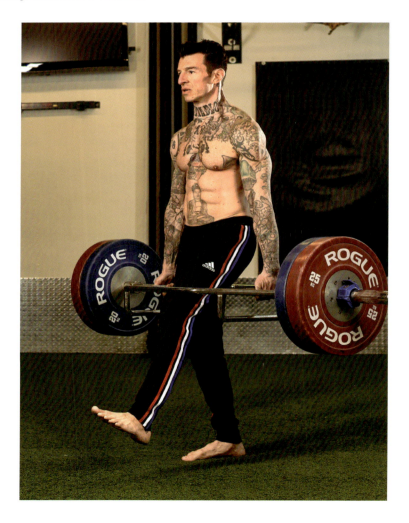

SHOULDER STRETCH #1
POLE ASSISTED

1 - Stand up and place your arm straight out, so that it is parallel to the ground.

2 - Place the hand of your extended arm against a pole or wall, pressing it against the surface and rotate your body away. Use the pole for leverage.

3 - Hold this position and repeat on the opposite side.

Works: Anterior deltoids, pectorals.

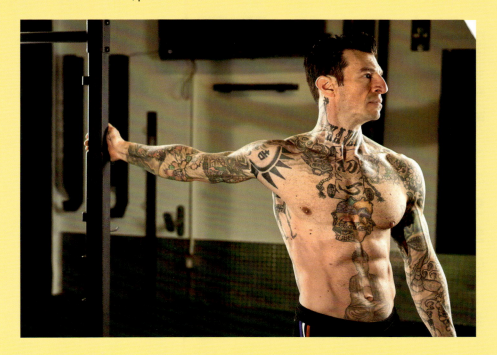

SHOULDER STRETCH #2
BAR ASSISTED

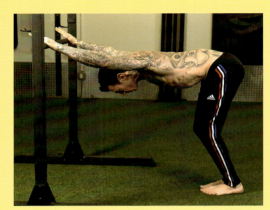

1 - Grasp a bar of approximately waist height slightly wider than shoulder width, using an overhand grip. Bend your knees and hips so that your torso is almost parallel to the ground; maintain a slight arch in your back.

2 - Keep your arms straight and press your chest down, without tucking your chin or rounding your back forward.

3 - Breathe slowly, press down as you exhale and return to the starting position.

Works: Deltoids, pectorals, biceps brachii, latissimus dorsi.

SHOULDER STRETCH #3
CAMEL

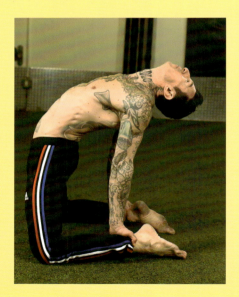

1 - Kneel down, lift your chest up and lean back. Put your hands on your lower back and walk them down until they are above your ankles with the thumbs pointed out.

2 - Push your hips forward and lift your chest and throat as high and far back as you can.

3 - Hold and then reverse the movement to return to the starting position.

Works: Pectorals, anterior deltoids, abdominals, hip flexors, spinal erectors.

ARMS

1. Barbell Curl
2. Dumbbell Curl
3. Bodyweight Curl
4. Bench Dip
5. Dip
6. Weighted Dip
7. Single Bar Dip
8. Barbell Skullcrusher
9. Bodyweight Skullcrusher
10. Arm Stretches

BARBELL CURL

The curl is a secondary exercise. It is an excellent complement to the larger movements that recruit more (or bigger) muscles and yield greater energy expenditure. Curls are a great finisher.

1 - Stand up straight with your feet flat on the floor and your body braced. Hold a barbell approximately shoulder width using an underhand grip.

2 - Keep your elbows against your sides and bend them, curling the bar toward your chest.

3 - Pause briefly before lowering the bar back to the starting position.

Trainer Talk: Try to lift from your arms only, without using any momentum or swinging the bar.

Primary Muscles: Biceps, brachialis.

Secondary Muscles: N/A

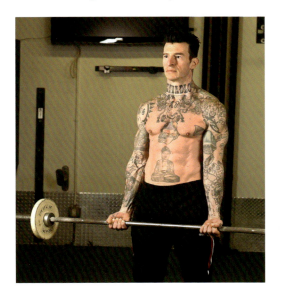
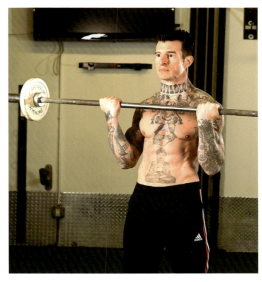

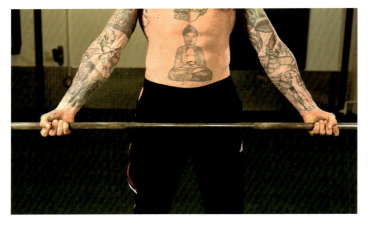

A wider hand position places greater emphasis on the shorter, inner head of the biceps as well as the brachialis, giving the biceps greater thickness.

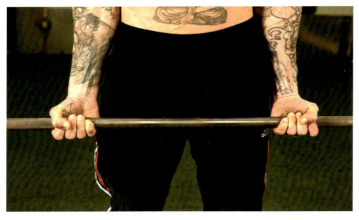

A close grip targets the longer, outer head, giving a greater "peak".

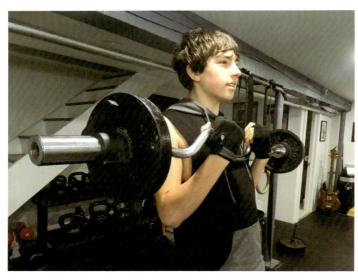

For those who experience stress in their wrists or elbows, the E-Z bar is a great option.

DUMBBELL CURL

When using dumbbells, each arm functions on its own without being fixed to the other. Because of this, you must employ more stabilizer muscles and can achieve a more natural range-of-motion.

1 - Stand up straight with your feet flat on the floor and your body braced. Hold a dumbbell in each hand using a parallel (neutral) grip.

2 - Keep your elbows against your sides and bend them, curling the dumbbells toward your chest. Allow your arm to rotate at the shoulder into an underhand grip.

3 - Pause briefly before lowering the bar back to the starting position.

Trainer Talk: Dumbbell curls can be performed standing or seated on a bench. Standing calls for more core recruitment, as the bench provides more stability. You may also keep your hands in a parallel grip, without rotating. This is called a "hammer curl".

Primary Muscles: Biceps, brachialis.

Secondary Muscles: N/A

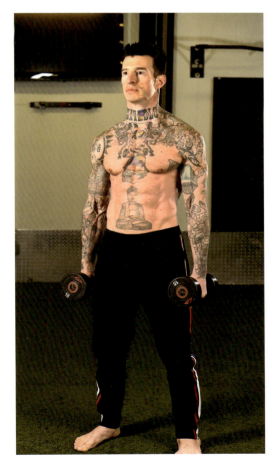 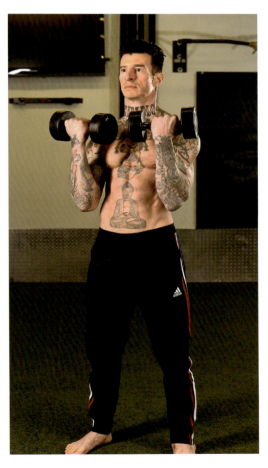

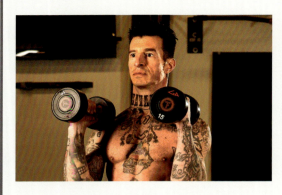

HAMMER CURL

"Hammer" dumbbell curls involve keeping the dumbbells in a parallel (neutral) grip, with your palms facing each other, for the entire range of motion. This position is generally easy on the elbow joints and places greater emphasis on the brachialis.

BODYWEIGHT CURL

This curl variation requires a greater degree of full body muscular engagement than the others. Bodyweight curls work well with gymnastics rings or suspension trainers.

1 - Grasp a set of rings with your palms facing up and your arms straight in front of you. Walk your feet forward, bend your elbows and extend your legs. Keep your feet together and form a straight line from your head to your heels.

2 - Bend at the elbows and wrists only, without moving your shoulders and curl the rings toward your forehead. Make sure that your arms remain perpendicular to your torso the whole time. Do not let your elbows flare out to the sides.

3 - Pause briefly when the rings almost touch your head. Lower yourself back to the starting position.

Trainer Talk: The bodyweight curl can also be performed with your feet flat on the floor and your knees bent. Doing so provides a more solid footing.

Primary Muscles: Biceps, brachialis.

Secondary Muscles: Abdominals, glutes, latissimus dorsi.

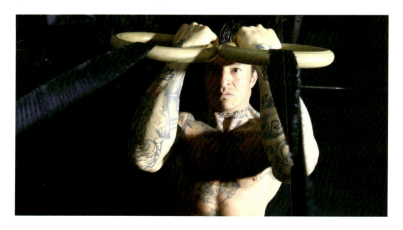

BENCH DIP

Performing dips with your feet on the ground places less of your body weight in your arms than a traditional dip does.

1 - Place your hands shoulder width apart on a bench behind you. Keep your feet together on the ground and your legs straight.

2 - With your chest and chin up, bend your elbows and shoulders to lower your hips toward the ground.

3 - Pause briefly at the bottom, then press yourself back to the starting position.

Trainer Talk: The bench dip can also be performed with your feet flat on the floor and your knees bent. Doing so decreases the difficulty of the exercise.

Primary Muscles: Triceps, pectorals.

Secondary Muscles: Anterior deltoids.

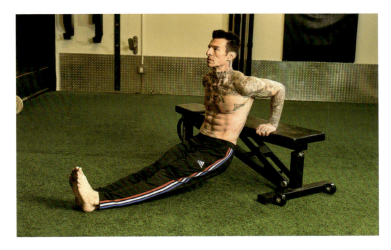

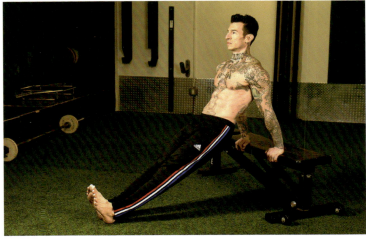

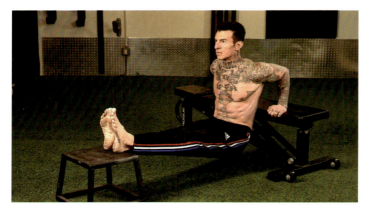

Elevating your feet places a greater amount of weight into your arms than a standard bench dip does, but still not as much as a traditional dip. The higher you place your feet, the more difficult the exercise becomes. Start with a low step.

DIP

The dip is a calisthenics classic. It is one of the finest measures of relative strength and one of my personal favorite exercises.

1 - Position yourself upright between two parallel bars. Grasp the bars and lock your elbows. Keep your feet off the floor.

2 - With your chest and chin up, bend your elbows and shoulders to lower yourself toward the ground.

3 - Pause briefly at the bottom, then press yourself back to the starting position.

Trainer Talk: Make sure your elbows point behind you and do not flare out to the sides. This will keep tension on your triceps and minimize shearing in your shoulder joints.

Primary Muscles: Triceps, pectorals.

Secondary Muscles: Anterior deltoids, abdominals.

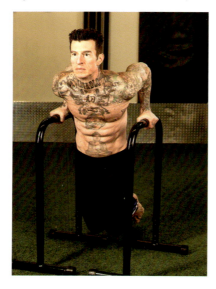
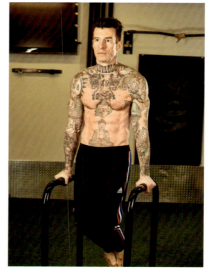

PROTECT YOUR NECK

It is important to maintain space between your shoulders and ears when performing dips. Shrugged shoulders in this position are poor for upper spinal health and render the exercise less effective.

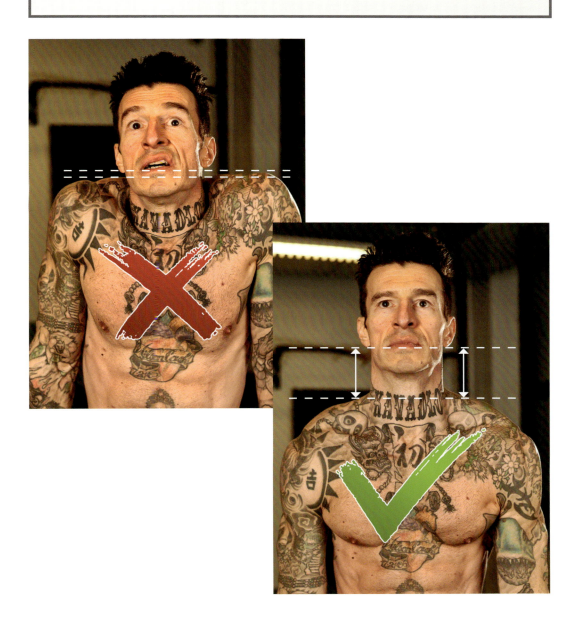

WEIGHTED DIP

Adding external resistance to this bodyweight classic is an excellent way to train harder, employ more of your core and trigger greater muscular growth, without having to incorporate a different movement pattern. A weighted belt, vest or chain work well for weighted dips.

1 - Affix the weight to your body so that it is evenly distributed and does not swing. Position yourself upright between two parallel bars. Grasp the bars and lock your elbows. Keep your feet off the floor.

2 - With your chest and chin up, bend your elbows and shoulders to lower yourself to the ground.

3 - Pause briefly at the bottom, then press yourself back to the starting position.

Trainer Talk: Weighted dips can potentially place a lot of stress on the elbows. If you have elbow issues or are recovering from an injury, it may be best to avoid weighted dips.

Primary Muscles: Triceps, pectorals.

Secondary Muscles: Anterior deltoids, abdominals.

CAUTION! Do not attempt this exercise until you are proficient with unweighted dips. Progress slowly.

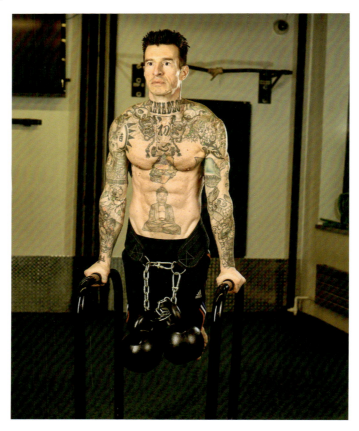

SINGLE BAR DIP

Rather than descend between two bars (as in a standard dip), the single bar dip (aka straight bar dip) compels you to maneuver around only one bar. It is an excellent lead up step to the muscle-up.

1 - Position yourself upright in front of a bar that is higher than your waist. Grasp the bar and lock your elbows. You may have to jump into this position. Keep your feet off the floor.

2 - With your chest and chin up, bend your elbows and shoulders to lower your chest as close to the bar as possible. Because your hands will be in front of you, it is helpful to extend your legs in front and use them as a counterweight to your upper body.

3 - Pause briefly at the bottom, then press yourself back to the starting position.

Trainer Talk: Make sure your elbows point behind you and do not flare out to the sides. This will keep tension on your triceps and minimize shearing in your shoulder joints.

Primary Muscles: Triceps, pectorals.

Secondary Muscles: Anterior deltoids, abdominals, forearms.

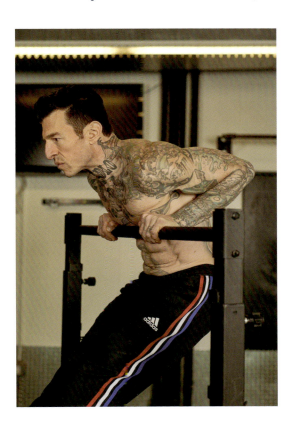
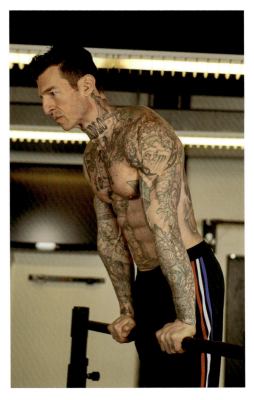

BARBELL SKULLCRUSHER

The skullcrusher is a lying triceps extension. The bench provides stability and keeps the focus on the triceps.

1 - Lie down on a bench with your feet flat on the floor and your body braced. Place your hands on the bar shoulder width apart or slightly closer. Extend your arms.

2 - Bend at the elbows and wrists only, without moving your shoulders and lower the bar toward your forehead.

3 - Pause briefly when the bar almost touches your head and press the bar back to starting position.

Trainer Talk: Make sure your elbows do not flare out to the sides. An E-Z bar also works well for this exercise.

Primary Muscles: Triceps.

Secondary Muscles: Anterior deltoids, forearms.

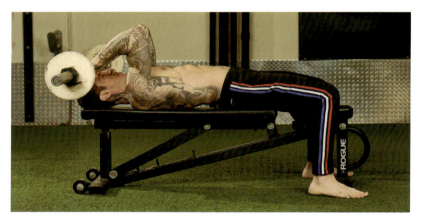

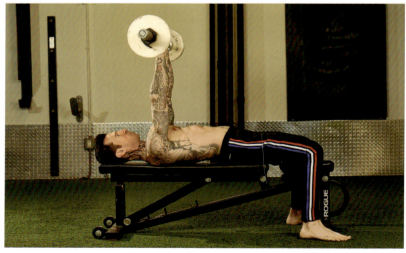

BODYWEIGHT SKULLCRUSHER

The bodyweight skullcrusher is a calisthenics version of the traditional weight training exercise. This variant requires much greater core recruitment.

1 - Place your hands on a bench or bar shoulder width apart or slightly closer. Keep your feet together on the ground and form a straight line from your head to your heels.

2 - Bend at the elbows and wrists only, without moving your shoulders, and lower your forehead toward the bench.

3 - Pause briefly when your head almost touches the bench. Press yourself back to the starting position.

Trainer Talk: The higher you place your hands, the more forgiving the exercise becomes. Beginners will want to use a very high bench. Make sure your elbows point behind you and do not flare out to the sides. Gymnastics rings or suspension trainers also work well for this exercise.

Primary Muscles: Triceps.

Secondary Muscles: Anterior deltoids, forearms, abdominals, pectorals.

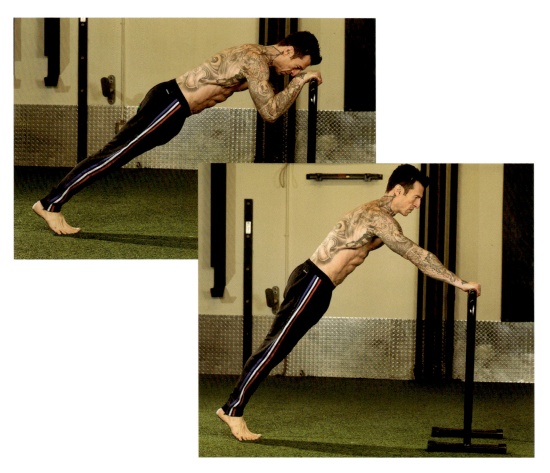

ON FOREARMS

There are no forearm specific exercises in this book. We spoke of primary exercises (deadlift or pull-up for example) and secondary exercises (lat raise or dumbbell curl for example). Forearm-specific exercises would be tertiary. Exercises like pull-ups, deadlifts, hanging abs and carrys work your forearms intensely. Forearm isolation-style exercises do exist, but they are not part of this program. There are more efficient ways to spend your time in the gym.

ARM STRETCH #1
BICEPS

1 - Stand up tall, lift your chest and extend your arm in front of you.

2 - Lock your elbow and use your other hand to bend your hand back at the wrist. Make sure your fingers are pointing down.

3 - Keep your arm straight and hold. Repeat on the opposite side.

Works: Biceps, brachialis.

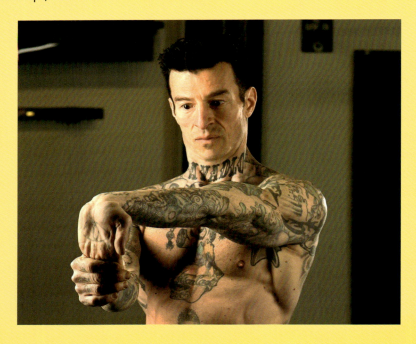

HYBRID STRENGTH TRAINING

ARM STRETCH #2
TRICEPS

1 - Stand up tall, lift your chest and bring your arm up and behind your head, bend at the elbow.

2 - Use your other arm to grab the elbow and gently press deeper into the stretch.

3 - Keep your chin up and hold. Repeat on the opposite side.

Works: Triceps, latissimus dorsi, medial deltoids.

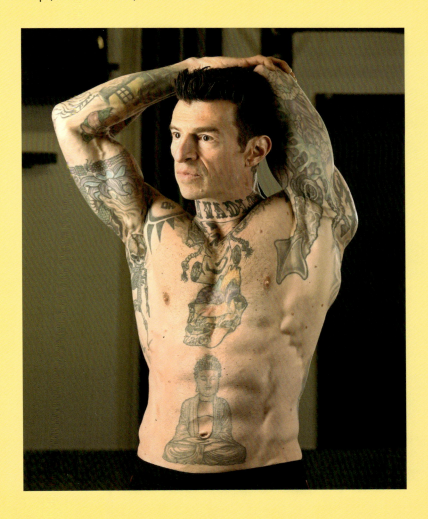

ARM STRETCH #3
FOREARM

1 - Make a tight fist and grab your wrist snugly with your other hand.

2 - In a deliberate and exaggerated motion, slowly rotate your wrist several times.

3 - Rotate your wrist in both directions, then repeat on the opposite side.

Works: Forearms.

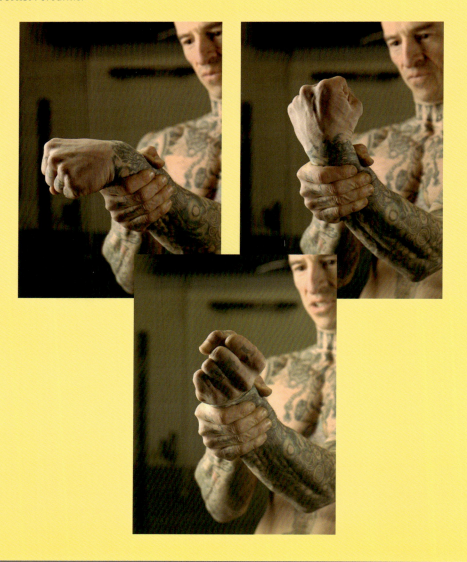

HYBRID STRENGTH TRAINING

ABS

1. Sit-up
2. Crossover Sit-up
3. Knee Tuck
4. Bent Leg Raise
5. Straight Leg Raise
6. Seated Knee Raise
7. Jackknife Sit-up
8. Hanging Knee Raise
9. Crossover Hanging Knee Raise
10. Hanging Leg Raise
11. Crossover Hanging Leg Raise
12. Abs Stretches

SIT-UP

The sit-up is a calisthenics classic. Many fads have come and gone but sit-ups are timeless.

1 - Lie on the ground with your knees up and both feet flat on the floor. Place your hands behind your head or your arms across your chest.

2 - Squeeze with your abs until your upper body comes all the way up toward your knees, curling from the abdomen.

3 - Pause briefly, then lower yourself back down to the starting position.

Trainer Talk: Make sure you initiate the movement from your abs, not your neck or shoulders. It may be helpful at the beginning to stabilize your feet under an object or with a partner.

Primary Muscles: Abdominals.

Secondary Muscles: N/A

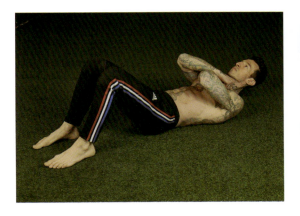
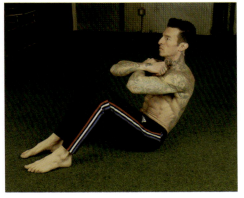

CROSSOVER SIT-UP

The crossover (aka sit-up with a twist) is a sit-up variant that incorporates trunk rotation to target the obliques more extensively.

1 - Lie on the ground with your knees up and both feet flat on the floor. Pick up one leg and place it across the other in a figure 4 position. Place one hand behind your head and the other by your side.

2 - Squeeze your abs in the direction of your bent knee, until your upper body comes up off the floor. Twist your bent elbow toward your bent knee, keeping your opposite shoulder flat on the ground.

3 - Pause briefly, then lower back down to the starting position. Complete your set in its entirety and then repeat on the opposite side.

Trainer Talk: Make sure you rotate your entire trunk, not just move the elbow. The shoulder blade must come off the ground.

Primary Muscles: Abdominals, obliques.

Secondary Muscles: N/A

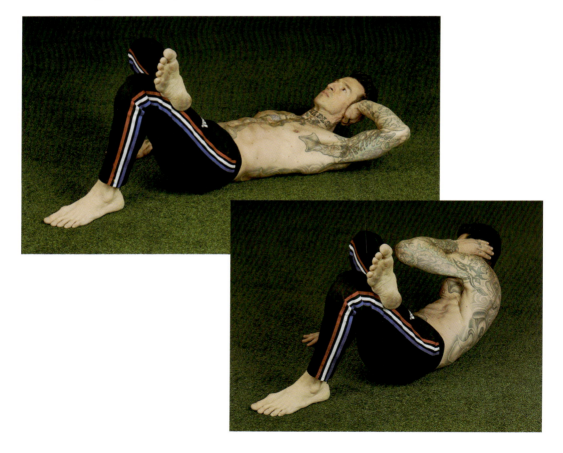

Knee Tuck

This calisthenics staple puts emphasis on the lower abdomen. Lying knee tucks teach you to curl from the abs and tilt the pelvis, which is important for every exercise moving forward.

1 - Lie on your back with your hands at your sides and your legs extended. Lift your heels and press your lower back into the ground.

2 - Keep your legs together and pull your knees toward your chest, bending at your knees.

3 - Extend your legs back out without letting your heels touch the floor.

Trainer Talk: Make sure you maintain contact between the ground and your lower back the entire time. You may tuck your chin to bring forth more tension.

Primary Muscles: Abdominals.

Secondary Muscles: Hip flexors.

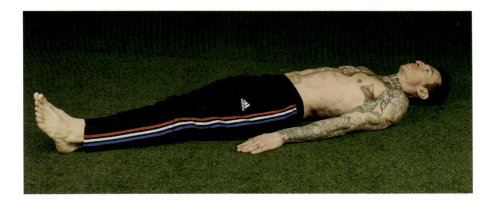

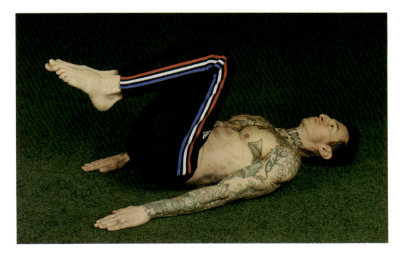

BENT LEG RAISE

This is an easier version of the following straight leg raise. The legs can be bent to infinite degrees, in order to regress the exercise if necessary.

1 - Lie on your back with your hands at your sides, your knees bent and your feet flat on the ground.

2 - Keep your legs together, with your knees bent. Hinge at the hip and raise your bent legs off the ground.

3 - Pause briefly, then lower your legs back to the starting position.

Trainer Talk: Bending your knees to a greater degree makes this exercise easier. Maintaining less of a knee bend makes it more difficult.

Primary Muscles: Abdominals.

Secondary Muscles: Hip flexors.

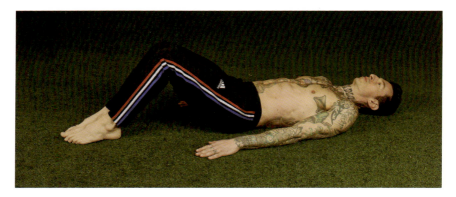

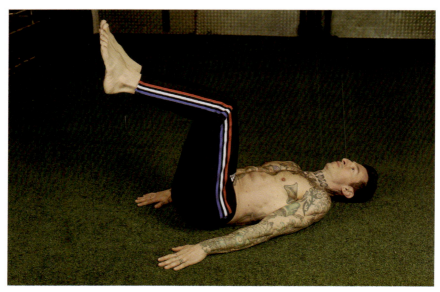

STRAIGHT LEG RAISE

This is a harder version of the bent leg raise because in this exercise, your legs remain completely straight the whole time, providing the most difficult leverage.

1 - Lie on your back with your hands at your sides and your legs extended.

2 - Keep your legs together and straight. Bend at the hips and raise your legs until they are perpendicular to the ground.

3 - Pause briefly, then lower your legs back to the starting position.

Trainer Talk: If you have discomfort in your lower back, then placing a small towel or your hands underneath can help to alleviate it.

Primary Muscles: Abdominals.

Secondary Muscles: Hip flexors.

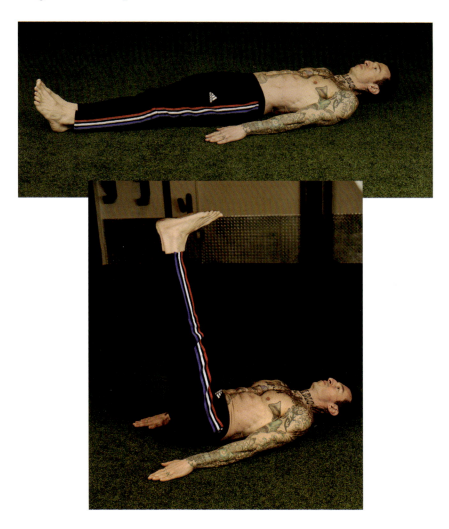

SEATED KNEE RAISE

This exercise is an excellent transitional step, as well as a viable exercise in its own right. Seated knee raises provide less stability than floor abs exercises but more than hanging abs.

1 - Sit on the edge of a bench with your legs extended in front of you.

2 - Keep your legs together and pull your knees toward your chest, bending at your knees.

3 - Pause briefly, then return to the starting position, without letting your feet touch the floor.

Trainer Talk: It may be helpful to clasp the side of the bench with your hands if you are new to this exercise.

Primary Muscles: Abdominals.

Secondary Muscles: Hip flexors.

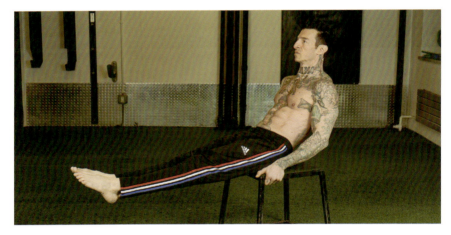

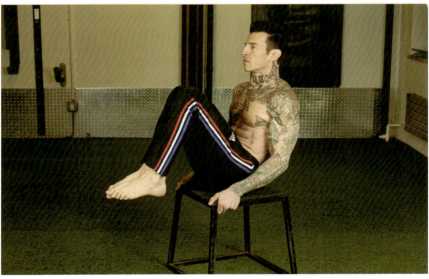

JACKKNIFE SIT-UP

Jackknife sit-ups target both the upper and lower abdomen.

1 - Lie on your back with your arms straight overhead and your legs extended.

2 - Bend at the hip and raise your legs until they are perpendicular to the ground, while sitting up at the same time, with your hands overhead. Your hands and feet should meet at the top contraction.

3 - Pause briefly, then return to the starting position.

Trainer Talk: Make sure you maintain contact between the ground and your lower back the entire time. Like any sit-up motion, be careful not to lead with your neck, but rather, curl from the abdominals.

Primary Muscles: Abdominals.

Secondary Muscles: Hip flexors.

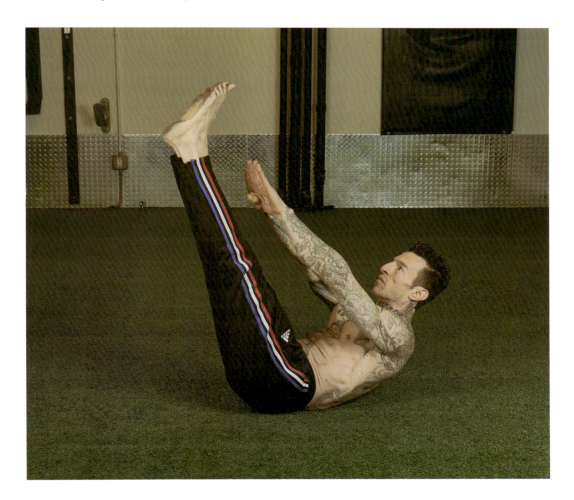

HANGING KNEE RAISE

Hanging knee raises (and all abs exercises on a bar) are more challenging than abs exercises performed on the floor. This is because the only points of contact are your hands and the leverage is less favorable.

1 - Grasp an overhead bar in an active hang (see sidebar on page 76) with your palms facing away from you

2 - Lift your knees toward your chest, tilting your pelvis slightly forward at the top in order to fully engage your abdominals.

3 - Pause briefly, then return to the starting position..

Trainer Talk: Keep your heels slightly in front of you in the bottom position in order to maintain abdominal tension.

Primary Muscles: Abdominals.

Secondary Muscles: Latissimus dorsi, rhomboids, serratus anterior, forearms.

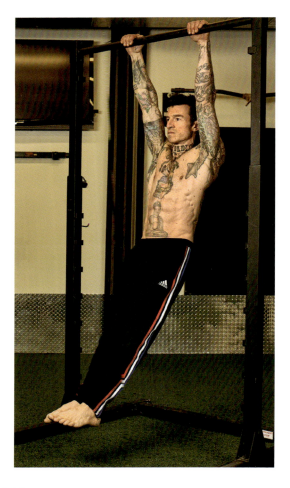
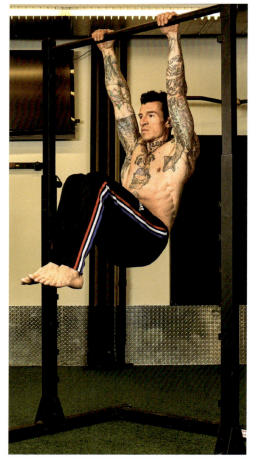

CROSSOVER HANGING KNEE RAISE

The crossover hanging knee raise (aka hanging knee raise with a twist) is a knee raise variant that incorporates trunk rotation to target the obliques more extensively.

1 - Grasp an overhead bar in an active hang (see sidebar on page 76) with your palms facing away from you.

2 - Lift your knees toward your armpit, tilting your pelvis forward and twisting at the top in order to fully engage your abdominals.

3 - Pause briefly, then return to the starting position and repeat on the other side. Alternate sides during your set, rather than completing one side in its entirety.

Trainer Talk: Do your best to avoid momentum with this exercise. Squeeze the bar tightly to maintain control.

Primary Muscles: Abdominals, obliques.

Secondary Muscles: Latissimus dorsi, rhomboids, serratus anterior, forearms.

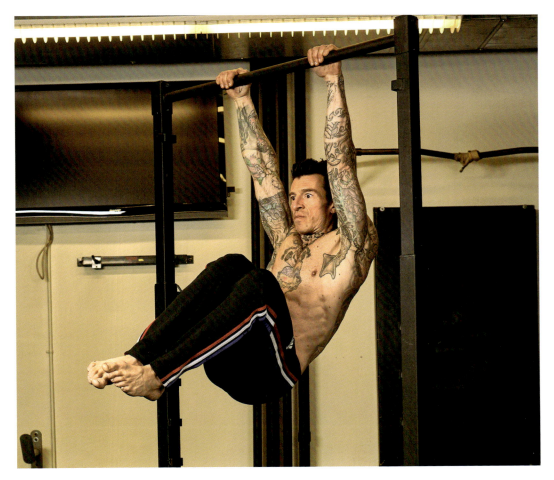

Hanging Leg Raise

This is a harder version of the hanging knee raise. The legs remain totally straight the whole time, providing the most difficult leverage.

1 - Grasp an overhead bar in an active hang (see sidebar on page 76) with your palms facing away from you.

2 - Keep your knees locked and lift your legs up, tilting your pelvis forward, until your legs are parallel to the ground. Flex your quadriceps in order to maintain straight legs the entire time.

3 - Pause briefly, then return to the starting position..

Trainer Talk: You can increase the difficulty of this exercise by bringing your legs all the way to the bar.

Primary Muscles: Abdominals.

Secondary Muscles: Latissimus dorsi, rhomboids, serratus anterior, forearms.

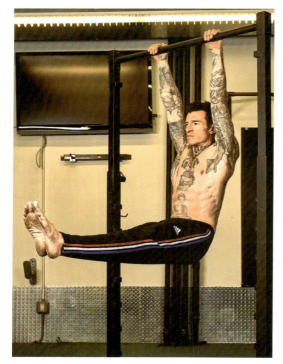

Parallel.

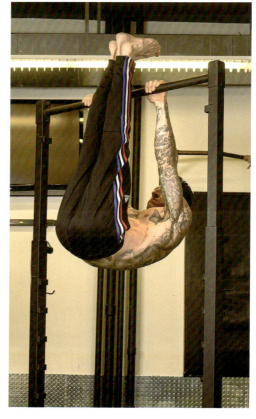

Legs to bar.

CROSSOVER HANGING LEG RAISE

The crossover hanging leg raise (aka hanging leg raise with a twist) is a leg raise variant that incorporates trunk rotation to target the obliques.

1 - Grasp an overhead bar in an active hang (see sidebar on page 76) with your palms facing away from you.

2 - Keep your knees locked and lift your legs up and to the side, tilting your pelvis forward, until your legs come in contact with the bar.

3 - Pause briefly, then return to the starting position and repeat on the other side. Alternate sides during your set, rather than completing one side in its entirety.

Trainer Talk: Squeeze your legs and feet together in order to generate more tension.

Primary Muscles: Abdominals, obliques.

Secondary Muscles: Latissimus dorsi, rhomboids, serratus anterior, forearms.

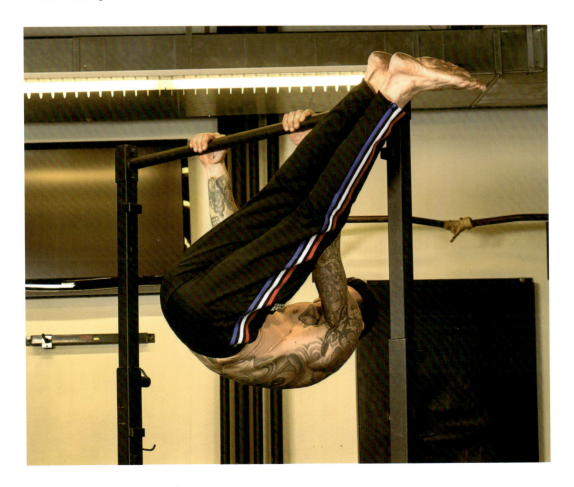

ABS STRETCH #1
LOW ABS STRETCH

1 - Start out at the bottom of a split-squat position with both knees bent to about 90°. Place your rear knee on the ground behind you and your forward foot flat on the floor. Engage your glutes for more stability.

2 - Lean forward, keeping your torso up, bending back the hip flexor and allowing your knee to get farther behind you as you stretch.

3 - Hold for several breaths. Repeat on the opposite side.

Works: Hip flexors, abdominals, quadriceps.

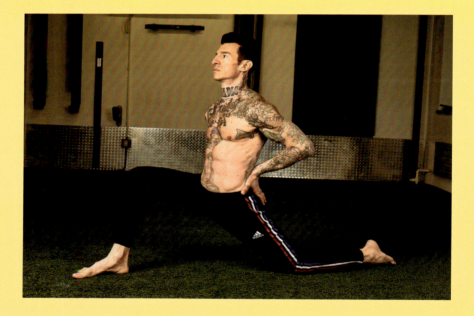

ABS STRETCH #2
BABY COBRA

1 - Lie facedown on the ground with your hands flat on the floor, thumbs by your armpits and elbows pointing up.

2 - Lift your chin, open your chest and extend your upper back to pick your head and chest off the floor. Aim to look at the ceiling. Pull your chest up with your back muscles and drive your hips down, rather than just pressing your hands into the ground.

3 - Keep your chin up and hold.

Works: Abdominals, pectorals.

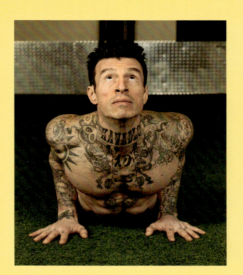

ABS STRETCH #3
SEATED TWIST

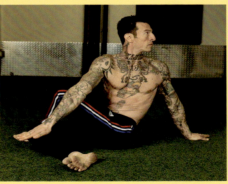

1 - Sit on the ground and cross one leg over the other, bending at the knee. Reach over with the opposite arm and place it against your knee, pushing your chest out and twisting your trunk toward and past the bent knee. Turn your head and look over your shoulder.

2 - Make sure you have your left hand and foot pressed flat on the ground when twisting to the left and your right foot pressed flat when twisting to the right.

3 - Keep your back straight and your chest high. Hold this for several breaths. Repeat on the opposite side.

Works: Abdominals, obliques, rhomboids, spinal erectors, pectorals.

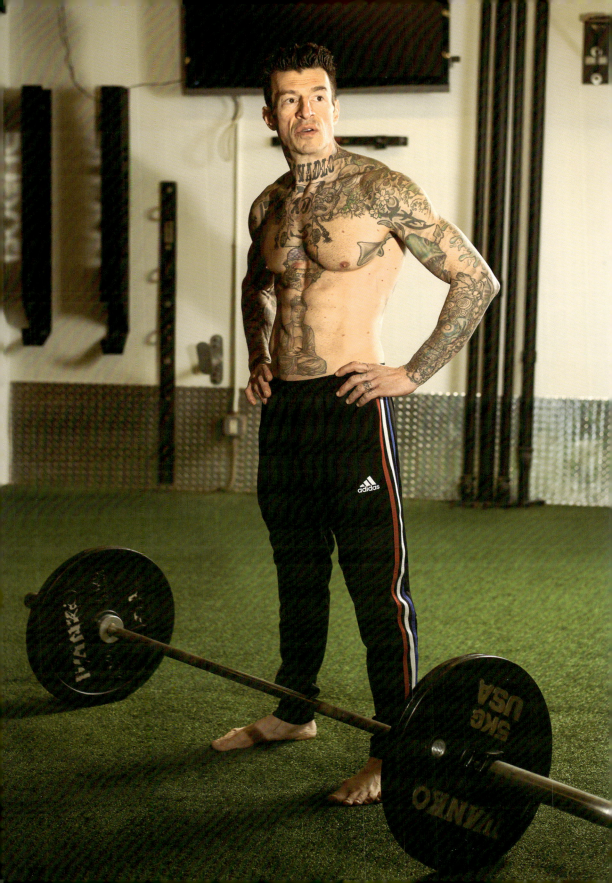

PART IV

PROGRAMS & PROGRAMMING

Now that you are familiar with the exercises, it's time to put them together. You know the moves. This is how you use them.

While it's always nice to have a plan on paper, it's the execution of the plan that matters. The programs that follow are composed as such because they work. But nothing will work if you won't, so show up excuse-free and ready to hit it hard. Refamiliarize yourself with the *Fundamentals of Strength Training* on page 11. Allocate time for your workouts and approach them with a clear mind.

What follows are three six-week Hybrid Strength Training programs:
- **BLUE FLAME (beginner to intermediate)**
- **RED HOT (intermediate to advanced)**
- **HELLYEAH! (advanced and beyond)**

Each one increases in difficulty from week to week through increased resistance, harder exercises and progressive rep schemes.

Every program is arranged in a clear, organized template, including warm-ups, sets/reps, alternative exercises and rest days. (Remember, "rest day" doesn't mean you avoid all activity. It's just a break in strength training, so please be as active as you want.) Each program concludes with a Self-Assessment. In order to know if you're ready for the next program, you must first see where you stand. These assessments consist of bodyweight baselines (based on number of reps) and barbell squats and deadlifts (based on one rep max). The assessments change from program to program.

The precise weight one can lift on any given exercise varies greatly from individual to individual. For that reason, the recommended resistances for the weighted exercises in these programs are categorized as *light weight (less than 50% of max lift), medium weight (50-80% of max lift) and heavy weight (greater than 80% of max lift)*. It would be impossible to list specific poundages that universally apply to all.

BLUE FLAME, RED HOT & HELLYEAH! are all about developing a powerful, shredded and amazingly strong body. Bonus workouts are also included, as well as additional information about programming.

On another note, not every exercise in this manual is included in these programs. That doesn't mean they're not valuable—simply that one cannot do everything at once. And while these programs are some of the most effective available, still be prepared to make changes if and when it's appropriate. Real and actionable strategies are important, but so is the ability to recalibrate. Whether that means swapping out an exercise, taking a longer rest period or modifying your grip, don't be afraid to adjust when called for. The only component you can't alter is your work ethic if you want results.

PROGRAM 1

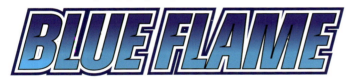

• This is a beginner to intermediate level six-week program consisting of three weekly workouts. Here's the split:

- **Day 1—Upper body**
- **Day 2—Lower body**
- **Day 3—Full body (Circuit)**

• The warm-ups consist of a series of stretches. Perform each one at least twice for a minimum 30 seconds.
• You may choose your rest days. While Days 1 and 2 may be done in succession, please take a rest day before and after Day 3.
• Work on mobility and get physical activity on your rest days.
• Assess yourself after six weeks.

PROGRAM 1
BLUE FLAME *WEEK 1*

DAY 1: CHEST, BACK, SHOULDERS
Warm-up: Pole assisted chest stretch, low squat semi-hang, double shoulder opener.

Exercise	Set	Rep	
Push-up	3	5 to 10	*•Perform all sets in sequence with 1-3 minutes rest in between.*
Overhead DB Press	3	5 to 10	*•Subsitute incline push-ups if push-ups are too difficult.*
One Arm DB Row (PER SIDE)	3	5 to 10	*•Use LIGHT WEIGHT for overhead press and one arm row.*
Bench Dip	3	5 to 10	
Active Bar Hang (IN SECONDS)	2	10	*•Perform bench dips with bent knees.*

DAY 2: LEGS, ABS
Warm-up: Quadriceps stretch, hip flexors stretch, hamstrings stretch.

Exercise	Set	Rep	
Bodyweight Squat	3	10	*•Perform all sets in sequence with 1-3 minutes rest in between.*
Goblet Squat	3	5 to 10	*•Use LIGHT WEIGHT for goblet squat.*
Hip Bridge	3	5 to 10	*•Keep your heels flat on the floor for all leg exercises.*
Sit-up	3	10	*•Keep your low back flat on the floor for all abs exercises.*

DAY 3: FULL BODY (CIRCUIT TRAINING)
Warm-up: Pole assisted chest stretch, low squat semi-hang, double shoulder opener, quadriceps stretch, hip flexors stretch, hamstrings stretch.

Exercise	Set	Rep	
Bodyweight Squat	2	10	*•This is a circuit.*
Push-up	2	5 to 10	*•Perform one set of each exercise in succession, with as little rest as possible in between.*
Active Bar Hang (IN SECONDS)	2	10	*•After you complete one set of each exercise, rest as long as you need.*
Bodyweight Split Squat (PER SIDE)	2	5 to 10	
Overhead DB Press	2	5 to 10	*•Perform your second set of each exercise in succession, with as little rest as possible in between.*
One arm DB Row (PER SIDE)	2	5 to 10	
Sit-up	2	10	

PROGRAM 1

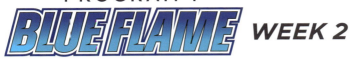 *WEEK 2*

DAY 1: CHEST, BACK, SHOULDERS
Warm-up: Pole assisted chest stretch, low squat semi-hang, double shoulder opener.

Exercise	Set	Rep	
Push-up	3	5 to 10	•Perform all sets in sequence with 1-3 minutes rest in between.
Overhead DB Press	3	5 to 10	•Substitute incline push-ups if push-ups are too difficult.
One Arm DB Row (PER SIDE)	3	5 to 10	•Use LIGHT WEIGHT for overhead press and one arm row.
Bench Dip	3	5 to 10	
Active Bar Hang (IN SECONDS)	2	10	•Perform bench dips with bent knees.

DAY 2: LEGS, ABS
Warm-up: Quadriceps stretch, hip flexors stretch, hamstrings stretch.

Exercise	Set	Rep	
Bodyweight Squat	3	10	•Perform all sets in sequence with 1-3 minutes rest in between.
Goblet Squat	3	5 to 10	•Use LIGHT WEIGHT for goblet squat.
Hip Bridge	3	5 to 10	•Keep your heels flat on the floor for all leg exercises.
Sit-up	3	10	•Keep your low back flat on the floor for all abs exercises.

DAY 3: FULL BODY (CIRCUIT TRAINING)
Warm-up: Pole assisted chest stretch, low squat semi-hang, double shoulder opener, quadriceps stretch, hip flexors stretch, hamstrings stretch.

Exercise	Set	Rep	
Bodyweight Squat	2	10	•This is a circuit.
Push-up	2	5 to 10	•Perform one set of each exercise in succession, with as little rest as possible in between.
Active Bar Hang (IN SECONDS)	2	10	
Bodyweight Split Squat (PER SIDE)	2	5 to 10	•After you complete one set of each exercise, rest as long as you need.
Overhead DB Press	2	5 to 10	•Perform your second set of each exercise in succession, with as little rest as possible in between.
One arm DB Row (PER SIDE)	2	5 to 10	
Sit-up	2	10	

BLUE FLAME *WEEK 3*

DAY 1: CHEST, BACK, SHOULDERS
Warm-up: Pole assisted chest stretch, low squat semi-hang, double shoulder opener.

Exercise	Set	Rep	
Push-up	3	10 to 15	•Perform all sets in sequence with 1-3 minutes rest in between.
Overhead DB Press	3	10 to 12	•Subsitute incline push-ups if push-ups are too difficult.
One Arm DB Row (PER SIDE)	3	10 to 12	•Use MEDIUM WEIGHT for overhead press and one arm row.
Bench Dip	3	10 to 12	
Active Bar Hang (IN SECONDS)	2	30	•Perform bench dips with bent knees or straight legs.
V Pull-up	2	3	

DAY 2: LEGS, ABS
Warm-up: Quadriceps stretch, hip flexors stretch, hamstrings stretch.

Exercise	Set	Rep	
Bodyweight Squat	3	10 to 20	•Perform all sets in sequence with 1-3 minutes rest in between.
Goblet Squat	3	10 to 15	•Use LIGHT WEIGHT for goblet squat.
Bodyweight Split Squat (PER SIDE)	3	10	•Keep your heels flat on the floor for all leg exercises.
Hip Bridge	3	10	•Keep your low back flat on the floor for all abs exercises.
Sit-up	3	15	

DAY 3: FULL BODY (CIRCUIT TRAINING)
Warm-up: Pole assisted chest stretch, low squat semi-hang, double shoulder opener, quadriceps stretch, hip flexors stretch, hamstrings stretch.

Exercise	Set	Rep	
Bodyweight Squat	2	10 to 20	•This is a circuit.
Push-up	2	10 to 15	•Perform one set of each exercise in succession, with as little rest as possible in between.
V Pull-up	2	3	
Bodyweight Split Squat (PER SIDE)	2	10	•After you complete one set of each exercise, rest as long as you need.
Overhead DB Press	2	10 to 12	•Perform your second set of each exercise in succession, with as little rest as possible in between.
One arm DB Row (PER SIDE)	2	10 to 12	
Sit-up	2	15	

PROGRAM 1

BLUE FLAME — WEEK 4

DAY 1: CHEST, BACK, SHOULDERS
Warm-up: Pole assisted chest stretch, low squat semi-hang, double shoulder opener.

Exercise	Set	Rep	
Push-up	3	10 to 15	•Perform all sets in sequence with 1-3 minutes rest in between.
Overhead DB Press	3	10 to 12	•Subsitute incline push-ups if push-ups are too difficult.
One Arm DB Row (PER SIDE)	3	10 to 12	•Use MEDIUM WEIGHT for overhead press and one arm row.
Bench Dip	3	10 to 12	
Active Bar Hang (IN SECONDS)	2	30	•Perform bench dips with bent knees or straight legs.
V Pull-up	2	3	

DAY 2: LEGS, ABS
Warm-up: Quadriceps stretch, hip flexors stretch, hamstrings stretch.

Exercise	Set	Rep	
Bodyweight Squat	3	10 to 20	•Perform all sets in sequence with 1-3 minutes rest in between.
Goblet Squat	3	10 to 15	•Use LIGHT WEIGHT for goblet squat.
Bodyweight Split Squat (PER SIDE)	3	10	•Keep your heels flat on the floor for all leg exercises.
Hip Bridge	3	10	•Keep your low back flat on the floor for all abs exercises.
Sit-up	3	15	

DAY 3: FULL BODY (CIRCUIT TRAINING)
Warm-up: Pole assisted chest stretch, low squat semi-hang, double shoulder opener, quadriceps stretch, hip flexors stretch, hamstrings stretch.

Exercise	Set	Rep	
Bodyweight Squat	2	10 to 20	•This is a circuit.
Push-up	2	10 to 15	•Perform one set of each exercise in succession, with as little rest as possible in between.
V Pull-up	2	3	
Bodyweight Split Squat (PER SIDE)	2	10	•After you complete one set of each exercise, rest as long as you need.
Overhead DB Press	2	10 to 12	•Perform your second set of each exercise in succession, with as little rest as possible in between.
One arm DB Row (PER SIDE)	2	10 to 12	
Sit-up	2	15	

BLUE FLAME *WEEK 5*

DAY 1: CHEST, BACK, SHOULDERS
Warm-up: Pole assisted chest stretch, low squat semi-hang, double shoulder opener.

Exercise	Set	Rep	
Push-up	3	15 to 20	•Perform all sets in sequence with 1-3 minutes rest in between.
Barbell Bench Press	3	8 to 10	•Use LIGHT WEIGHT for barbell bench press.
Overhead DB Press	3	10 to 12	•Subsitute dumbbells if barbell bench press causes excessive discomfort.
One Arm DB Row (PER SIDE)	3	10 to 12	•Use MEDIUM to HEAVY WEIGHT for overhead press and one arm row.
Bench Dip	3	12 to 15	
V Pull-up	2	5	•Perform bench dips with bent knees or straight legs.
Chin-up	2	1 to 2	

DAY 2: LEGS, ABS
Warm-up: Quadriceps stretch, hip flexors stretch, hamstrings stretch.

Exercise	Set	Rep	
Bodyweight Squat	2	20 to 30	•Perform all sets in sequence with 1-3 minutes rest in between.
Goblet Squat	3	15	•Use MEDIUM WEIGHT for goblet squat and weighted split squat.
Weighted Split Squat (PER SIDE)	3	10	
Hip Bridge	3	15	•Keep your heels flat on the floor for all leg exercises.
Sit-up	3	20	•Keep your low back flat on the floor for all abs exercises.
Knee Tuck	3	10	

DAY 3: FULL BODY (CIRCUIT TRAINING)
Warm-up: Pole assisted chest stretch, low squat semi-hang, double shoulder opener, quadriceps stretch, hip flexors stretch, hamstrings stretch.

Exercise	Set	Rep	
Bodyweight Squat	3	10 to 20	•This is a circuit.
Push-up	3	10 to 20	•Perform one set of each exercise in succession, with as little rest as possible in between.
Chin-up	3	2	•After you complete one set of each exercise, rest as long as you need.
Sit-up	3	15	•Perform your second set of each exercise in succession, with as little rest as possible in between.
Weighted Split Squat (PER SIDE)	3	10	•After you complete your second set of each exercise, rest as long as you need.
Overhead DB Press	3	10 to 12	•Perform your third set of each exercise in succession, with as little rest as possible in between.
One arm DB Row (PER SIDE)	3	10 to 12	
Knee Tuck	3	10	

PROGRAM 1

BLUE FLAME WEEK 6

DAY 1: CHEST, BACK, SHOULDERS
Warm-up: Pole assisted chest stretch, low squat semi-hang, double shoulder opener.

Exercise	Set	Rep
Push-up	3	15 to 20
Barbell Bench Press	3	8 to 10
Overhead DB Press	3	10 to 12
One Arm DB Row (PER SIDE)	3	10 to 12
Bench Dip	3	12 to 15
V Pull-up	2	5
Chin-up	2	1 to 2

- Perform all sets in sequence with 1-3 minutes rest in between.
- Use LIGHT WEIGHT for barbell bench press.
- Subsitute dumbbells if barbell bench press causes excessive discomfort.
- Use MEDIUM to HEAVY WEIGHT for overhead press and one arm row.
- Perform bench dips with bent knees or straight legs.

DAY 2: LEGS, ABS
Warm-up: Quadriceps stretch, hip flexors stretch, hamstrings stretch.

Exercise	Set	Rep
Bodyweight Squat	2	20 to 30
Goblet Squat	3	15
Weighted Split Squat (PER SIDE)	3	10
Hip Bridge	3	15
Sit-up	3	20
Knee Tuck	3	10

- Perform all sets in sequence with 1-3 minutes rest in between.
- Use MEDIUM WEIGHT for goblet squat and weighted split squat.
- Keep your heels flat on the floor for all leg exercises.
- Keep your low back flat on the floor for all abs exercises.

DAY 3: FULL BODY (CIRCUIT TRAINING)
Warm-up: Pole assisted chest stretch, low squat semi-hang, double shoulder opener, quadriceps stretch, hip flexors stretch, hamstrings stretch.

Exercise	Set	Rep
Bodyweight Squat	3	10 to 20
Push-up	3	10 to 20
Chin-up	3	2
Sit-up	3	15
Weighted Split Squat (PER SIDE)	3	10
Overhead DB Press	3	10 to 12
One arm DB Row (PER SIDE)	3	10 to 12
Knee Tuck	3	10

- This is a circuit.
- Perform one set of each exercise in succession, with as little rest as possible in between.
- After you complete one set of each exercise, rest as long as you need.
- Perform your second set of each exercise in succession, with as little rest as possible in between.
- After you complete your second set of each exercise, rest as long as you need.
- Perform your third set of each exercise in succession, with as little rest as possible in between.

BLUE FLAME

ASSESS YOURSELF

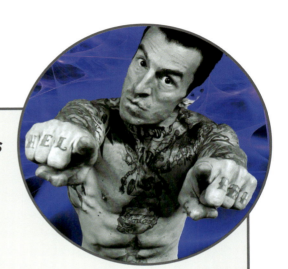

The following benchmarks serve as a measurable standard of achievement.

How do you measure up?

CAN YOU DO IT?

30 Squats	_____YES	_____NO
20 Push-ups	_____YES	_____NO
2 Chin-ups	_____YES	_____NO

- *If YES TO ALL THREE, then you may attempt RED HOT.*
- *If NO, then repeat the last 2 weeks of BLUE FLAME.*
- *If needed, add one day, specifically training the exercise(s) you did not complete.*

PROGRAM 2

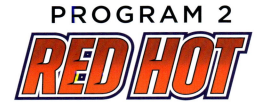

This is an intermediate to advanced level six-week program consisting of four weekly workouts. Here's the split:

- **Day 1—Upper body (Chest and back emphasis)**
- **Day 2—Lower body (Legs and abs)**
- **Day 3—Upper Body (Shoulders)**
- **Day 4—Upper body (Arms emphasis)**

- The warm-ups consist of a series of stretches and bodyweight exercises. Perform each stretch at least twice for a minimum 30 seconds. Do each exercise for at least 3 sets of 10.
- You may choose your rest days, but do not take more than two consecutively.
- Work on mobility and get physical activity on your rest days.
- Assess yourself after six weeks.

PROGRAM 2

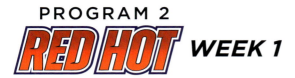 *WEEK 1*

DAY 1: CHEST, BACK, ARMS (CHEST & BACK CENTRIC)
Warm-up: Pole assisted chest stretch, low squat semi-hang, push-up, bodyweight row.

Exercise	Set	Rep	
Bench Press	3	10 to 12	•Perform all sets in sequence with 1-3 minutes rest in between.
Barbell Row	3	10 to 12	•Use LIGHT TO MEDIUM WEIGHT for barbell bench press and barbell row.
Chin-up	3	3 to 5	•Subsitute dumbbells if barbell bench press causes shoulder pain.
Pull-up	3	1 to 2	•Always do an unloaded barbell set before adding weight to bench press.
Dip	3	5 to 10	

DAY 2: LEGS, ABS
Warm-up: Quadriceps stretch, hip flexors stretch, hamstrings stretch, bodyweight squat.

Exercise	Set	Rep	
Bodyweight Split Squat	2	10 PER SIDE	•Perform all sets in sequence with 1-3 minutes rest in between.
Barbell Squat	3	10 to 12	•Use LIGHT TO MEDIUM WEIGHT for barbell squat and deadlift.
Hip Bridge	2	10	•Always do an unloaded barbell set before adding weight to barbell squat.
Deadlift	5	5	
Jacknife	3	10	

DAY 3: SHOULDERS
Warm-up: Double shoulder opener, pole assisted shoulder stretch.

Exercise	Set	Rep	
OH Barbell Press	3	10 to 12	•Perform all sets in sequence with 1-3 minutes rest in between.
Wall Handstand	2	30 SEC	•Use LIGHT TO MEDIUM WEIGHT for overheard barbell press.
Lateral Raise	3	10	•Use LIGHT WEIGHT for lateral, front and rear delt raise.
Front Raise	3	10	•Subsitute dumbbells if barbell overhead press causes shoulder pain.
Rear Deltoid Raise	3	10	•Always do an unloaded barbell set before adding weight to shoulder press.

DAY 4: CHEST, BACK, ARMS, ABS (ARMS CENTRIC)
Warm-up: Biceps stretch, triceps stretch, forearms stertch, crescent moon, low abs stretch, push-up.

Exercise	Set	Rep	
Chin-up	3	3 to 5	•Perform all sets in sequence with 1-3 minutes rest in between.
Dip	3	5 to 10	•Use LIGHT TO MEDIUM WEIGHT for curl and skullcrusher.
Barbell Curl	3	10 to 12	
Skullcrusher	3	10 to 12	
Jacknife	3	10	

PROGRAM 2

RED HOT WEEK 2

DAY 1: CHEST, BACK, ARMS (CHEST & BACK CENTRIC)
Warm-up: Pole assisted chest stretch, low squat semi-hang, push-up, bodyweight row.

Exercise	Set	Rep	
Bench Press	3	10 to 12	•Perform all sets in sequence with 1-3 minutes rest in between.
Barbell Row	3	10 to 12	•Use LIGHT TO MEDIUM WEIGHT for barbell bench press and barbell row.
Chin-up	3	3 to 5	•Subsitute dumbbells if barbell bench press causes shoulder pain.
Pull-up	3	1 to 2	•Always do an unloaded barbell set before adding weight to bench press.
Dip	3	5 to 10	

DAY 2: LEGS, ABS
Warm-up: Quadriceps stretch, hip flexors stretch, hamstrings stretch, bodyweight squat.

Exercise	Set	Rep	
Bodyweight Split Squat	2	10 PER SIDE	•Perform all sets in sequence with 1-3 minutes rest in between.
Barbell Squat	3	10 to 12	•Use LIGHT TO MEDIUM WEIGHT for barbell squat and deadlift.
Hip Bridge	2	10	•Always do an unloaded barbell set before adding weight to barbell squat.
Deadlift	5	5	
Jacknife	3	10	

DAY 3: SHOULDERS
Warm-up: Double shoulder opener, pole assisted shoulder stretch.

Exercise	Set	Rep	
OH Barbell Press	3	10 to 12	•Perform all sets in sequence with 1-3 minutes rest in between.
Wall Handstand	2	30 SEC	•Use LIGHT TO MEDIUM WEIGHT for overheard barbell press.
Lateral Raise	3	10	•Use LIGHT WEIGHT for lateral, front and rear delt raise.
Front Raise	3	10	•Subsitute dumbbells if barbell overhead press causes shoulder pain.
Rear Deltoid Raise	3	10	•Always do an unloaded barbell set before adding weight to shoulder press.

DAY 4: CHEST, BACK, ARMS, ABS (ARMS CENTRIC)
Warm-up: Biceps stretch, triceps stretch, forearms stertch, crescent moon, low abs stretch, push-up.

Exercise	Set	Rep	
Chin-up	3	3 to 5	•Perform all sets in sequence with 1-3 minutes rest in between.
Dip	3	5 to 10	•Use LIGHT TO MEDIUM WEIGHT for curl and skullcrusher.
Barbell Curl	3	10 to 12	
Skullcrusher	3	10 to 12	
Jacknife	3	10	

PROGRAM 2
RED HOT *WEEK 3*

DAY 1: CHEST, BACK, ARMS (CHEST & BACK CENTRIC)
Warm-up: Pole assisted chest stretch, low squat semi-hang, push-up, bodyweight row.

Exercise	Set	Rep	
Bench Press	3	10 to 12	•Perform all sets in sequence with 1-3 minutes rest in between.
Incine DB Press	3	10 to 12	•Use MEDIUM TO HEAVY WEIGHT for barbell bench press, incline DB press and barbell row.
Barbell Row	3	10 to 12	
Chin-up	3	4 to 6	•Subsitute dumbbells if barbell bench press causes shoulder pain.
Pull-up	3	2 to 4	•Always do an unloaded barbell set before adding weight to bench press.
Dip	3	10 to 12	

DAY 2: LEGS, ABS
Warm-up: Quadriceps stretch, hip flexors stretch, hamstrings stretch, bodyweight squat.

Exercise	Set	Rep	
Bulgarian Split Squat	2	10 PER SIDE	•Perform all sets in sequence with 1-3 minutes rest in between.
Barbell Squat	3	10 to 12	•Use MEDIUM TO HEAVY WEIGHT for barbell squat.
One Leg Hip Bridge	2	5 PER SIDE	•Use MEDIUM TO HEAVY WEIGHT for deadlift.
Deadlift	5	5	•Always do an unloaded barbell set before adding weight to barbell squat.
Jacknife	3	15	
Hanging Knee Raise	3	10	

DAY 3: SHOULDERS
Warm-up: Double shoulder opener, pole assisted shoulder stretch.

Exercise	Set	Rep	
OH Barbell Press	3	10 to 12	•Perform all sets in sequence with 1-3 minutes rest in between.
Wall Handstand	2	45 SEC	•Use MEDIUM TO HEAVY WEIGHT for overheard barbell press.
Lateral Raise	3	10 to 12	•Use LIGHT WEIGHT for Arnold press, lateral, front and rear delt raise.
Front Raise	3	10 to 12	•Use MEDIUM WEIGHT for Arnold press.
Rear Deltoid Raise	3	10 to 12	•Subsitute dumbbells if barbell overhead press causes shoulder pain.
Arnold Press	3	10 to 12	•Always do an unloaded barbell set before adding weight to shoulder press.

DAY 4: CHEST, BACK, ARMS, ABS (ARMS CENTRIC)
Warm-up: Biceps stretch, triceps stretch, forearms stertch, crescent moon, low abs stretch, push-up.

Exercise	Set	Rep	
Chin-up	3	4 to 6	•Perform all sets in sequence with 1-3 minutes rest in between.
Dip	3	2 to 4	•Use MEDIUM TO HEAVY WEIGHT for curl and skullcrusher.
Barbell Curl	3	10	•Use LIGHT TO MEDIUM WEIGHT for pullover.
Skullcrusher	3	10	
Dumbbell Curl	3	10 PER SIDE	
Pullover	3	10	
Jacknife	3	10	

PROGRAM 2

RED HOT *WEEK 4*

DAY 1: CHEST, BACK, ARMS (CHEST & BACK CENTRIC)
Warm-up: Pole assisted chest stretch, low squat semi-hang, push-up, bodyweight row.

Exercise	Set	Rep
Bench Press	3	10 to 12
Incine DB Press	3	10 to 12
Barbell Row	3	10 to 12
Chin-up	3	4 to 6
Pull-up	3	2 to 4
Dip	3	10 to 12

- Perform all sets in sequence with 1-3 minutes rest in between.
- Use MEDIUM TO HEAVY WEIGHT for barbell bench press, incline DB press and barbell row.
- Subsitute dumbbells if barbell bench press causes shoulder pain.
- Always do an unloaded barbell set before adding weight to bench press.

DAY 2: LEGS, ABS
Warm-up: Quadriceps stretch, hip flexors stretch, hamstrings stretch, bodyweight squat.

Exercise	Set	Rep
Bulgarian Split Squat	2	10 PER SIDE
Barbell Squat	3	10 to 12
One Leg Hip Bridge	2	5 PER SIDE
Deadlift	5	5
Jacknife	3	15
Hanging Knee Raise	3	10

- Perform all sets in sequence with 1-3 minutes rest in between.
- Use MEDIUM TO HEAVY WEIGHT for barbell squat.
- Use MEDIUM TO HEAVY WEIGHT for deadlift.
- Always do an unloaded barbell set before adding weight to barbell squat.

DAY 3: SHOULDERS
Warm-up: Double shoulder opener, pole assisted shoulder stretch.

Exercise	Set	Rep
OH Barbell Press	3	10 to 12
Wall Handstand	2	45 SEC
Lateral Raise	3	10 to 12
Front Raise	3	10 to 12
Rear Deltoid Raise	3	10 to 12
Arnold Press	3	10 to 12

- Perform all sets in sequence with 1-3 minutes rest in between.
- Use MEDIUM TO HEAVY WEIGHT for overheard barbell press.
- Use LIGHT WEIGHT for Arnold press, lateral, front and rear delt raise.
- Use MEDIUM WEIGHT for Arnold press.
- Subsitute dumbbells if barbell overhead press causes shoulder pain.
- Always do an unloaded barbell set before adding weight to shoulder press.

DAY 4: CHEST, BACK, ARMS, ABS (ARMS CENTRIC)
Warm-up: Biceps stretch, triceps stretch, forearms stertch, crescent moon, low abs stretch, push-up.

Exercise	Set	Rep
Chin-up	3	4 to 6
Dip	3	2 to 4
Barbell Curl	3	10
Skullcrusher	3	10
Dumbbell Curl	3	10 PER SIDE
Pullover	3	10
Jacknife	3	10

- Perform all sets in sequence with 1-3 minutes rest in between.
- Use MEDIUM TO HEAVY WEIGHT for curl and skullcrusher.
- Use LIGHT TO MEDIUM WEIGHT for pullover.

PROGRAM 2
RED HOT WEEK 5

DAY 1: CHEST, BACK, ARMS (CHEST & BACK CENTRIC)
Warm-up: Pole assisted chest stretch, low squat semi-hang, push-up, bodyweight row.

Exercise	Set	Rep
Bench Press	3	8 to 10
Incine DB Press	3	10 to 12
Barbell Row	3	8 to 10
One Arm DB Row	3	8 to 12 PER SIDE
Chin-up	3	5 to 7
Pull-up	3	3 to 5
Dip	3	12 to 15

- Perform all sets in sequence with 1-3 minutes rest in between.
- Work up to HEAVY WEIGHT for barbell bench press and barbell row.
- Use MEDIUM TO HEAVY WEIGHT for incline DB press and one arm DB row.
- Subsitute dumbbells if barbell bench press causes shoulder pain.
- Always do an unloaded barbell set before adding weight to bench press.

DAY 2: LEGS, ABS
Warm-up: Quadriceps stretch, hip flexors stretch, hamstrings stretch, bodyweight squat.

Exercise	Set	Rep
Weighted Bulgarian Split Squat	2	1 PER SIDE
Barbell Squat	3	8 to 10
One Leg Hip Bridge	2	10 PER SIDE
Deadlift	5	5
Jacknife	3	20
Hanging Knee Raise	3	15

- Perform all sets in sequence with 1-3 minutes rest in between.
- Work up to HEAVY WEIGHT for barbell squat.
- Work up to HEAVY WEIGHT for deadlift.
- Always do an unloaded barbell set before adding weight to barbell squat.

DAY 3: SHOULDERS
Warm-up: Double shoulder opener, pole assisted shoulder stretch.

Exercise	Set	Rep
OH Barbell Press	3	8 to 10
Wall Handstand	1	45 SEC
Handstand Push-up	2	1
Lateral Raise	3	15
Front Raise	3	15
Rear Deltoid Raise	3	15
Arnold Press	3	10 to 12

- Perform all sets in sequence with 1-3 minutes rest in between.
- Work up to HEAVY WEIGHT for overheard barbell press.
- Use LIGHT WEIGHT for lateral, front and rear delt raise.
- Use MEDIUM TO HEAVY WEIGHT for Arnold press.
- Subsitute dumbbells if barbell overhead press causes shoulder pain.
- Subsitute wall handstand if handstand push-ups are too difficult.
- Always do an unloaded barbell set before adding weight to shoulder press.

DAY 4: CHEST, BACK, ARMS, ABS (ARMS CENTRIC)
Warm-up: Biceps stretch, triceps stretch, forearms stertch, crescent moon, low abs stretch, push-up.

Exercise	Set	Rep
Chin-up	3	5 to 7
Pull-up	1	3 to 5
Dip	3	12 to 15
Barbell Curl	3	10
Skullcrusher	3	10
Dumbbell Curl (PER SIDE)	3	10
Pullover	3	10
Jacknife	3	20

- Perform all sets in sequence with 1-3 minutes rest in between.
- Work up to HEAVY WEIGHT for curl and skullcrusher.
- Use MEDIUM TO HEAVY WEIGHT for pullover.

PROGRAM 2
RED HOT *WEEK 6*

DAY 1: CHEST, BACK, ARMS (CHEST & BACK CENTRIC)
Warm-up: Pole assisted chest stretch, low squat semi-hang, push-up, bodyweight row.

Exercise	Set	Rep	
Bench Press	3	8 to 10	•Perform all sets in sequence with 1-3 minutes rest in between.
Incine DB Press	3	10 to 12	•Work up to HEAVY WEIGHT for barbell bench press and barbell row.
Barbell Row	3	8 to 10	•Use MEDIUM TO HEAVY WEIGHT for incline DB press and one arm DB row.
One Arm DB Row	3	8 to 12 PER SIDE	
Chin-up	3	5 to 7	•Subsitute dumbbells if barbell bench press causes shoulder pain.
Pull-up	3	3 to 5	•Always do an unloaded barbell set before adding weight to bench press.
Dip	3	12 to 15	

DAY 2: LEGS, ABS
Warm-up: Quadriceps stretch, hip flexors stretch, hamstrings stretch, bodyweight squat.

Exercise	Set	Rep	
Weighted Bulgarian Split Squat	2	10 PER SIDE	•Perform all sets in sequence with 1-3 minutes rest in between.
Barbell Squat	3	8 to 10	•Work up to HEAVY WEIGHT for barbell squat.
One Leg Hip Bridge	2	10 PER SIDE	•Work up to HEAVY WEIGHT for deadlift.
Deadlift	5	5	•Always do an unloaded barbell set before adding weight to barbell squat.
Jacknife	3	20	
Hanging Knee Raise	3	15	

DAY 3: SHOULDERS
Warm-up: Double shoulder opener, pole assisted shoulder stretch.

Exercise	Set	Rep	
OH Barbell Press	3	8 to 10	•Perform all sets in sequence with 1-3 minutes rest in between.
Wall Handstand	1	45 SEC	•Work up to HEAVY WEIGHT for overheard barbell press.
Handstand Push-up	2	1	•Use LIGHT WEIGHT for lateral, front and rear delt raise.
Lateral Raise	3	15	•Use MEDIUM TO HEAVY WEIGHT for Arnold press.
Front Raise	3	15	•Subsitute dumbbells if barbell overhead press causes shoulder pain.
Rear Deltoid Raise	3	15	•Subsitute wall handstand if handstand push-ups are too difficult.
Arnold Press	3	10 to 12	•Always do an unloaded barbell set before adding weight to shoulder press.

DAY 4: CHEST, BACK, ARMS, ABS (ARMS CENTRIC)
Warm-up: Biceps stretch, triceps stretch, forearms stertch, crescent moon, low abs stretch, push-up.

Exercise	Set	Rep	
Chin-up	3	5 to 7	•Perform all sets in sequence with 1-3 minutes rest in between.
Pull-up	1	3 to 5	•Work up to HEAVY WEIGHT for curl and skullcrusher.
Dip	3	12 to 15	•Use MEDIUM TO HEAVY WEIGHT for pullover.
Barbell Curl	3	10	
Skullcrusher	3	10	
Dumbbell Curl	3	10 PER SIDE	
Pullover	3	10	
Jacknife	3	20	

PROGRAM 2
RED HOT
ASSESS YOURSELF

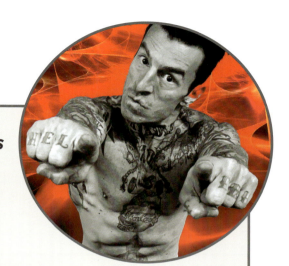

The following benchmarks serve as a measurable standard of achievement.

How do you measure up?

CAN YOU DO IT?

30 Push-ups   _____YES   _____NO

5 Pull-ups   _____YES   _____NO

Squat
  1x Bodyweight   _____YES   _____NO

Deadlift
  1.5x Bodyweight   _____YES   _____NO

- If YES TO ALL FOUR, then you may attempt *HELLYEAH!*
- If NO, then repeat the last 2 weeks of *RED HOT*.
- If needed, add one day, specifically training the exercise(s) you did not complete.

HYBRID STRENGTH TRAINING   147

PROGRAM 3

HELLYEAH! *WEEK 1*

•This is an advanced level six-week program consisting of five weekly workouts. Here's the split:

•**Day 1—Upper body**
•**Day 2—Lower body**
   (Deadlift emphasis)
•**Day 3—Upper body**
   (Calisthenics emphasis)

•**Day 4—Lower body**
   (Squat emphasis)
•**Day 5—Upper body**
   (Push/pull supersets)

•The warm-ups consist of a series of stretches and bodyweight exercises. Perform each stretch at least twice for a minimum 30 seconds. Do each exercise for at least 3 sets of 10.

•Take your first rest day between Day 2 and Day 3. You may choose your third rest day.

•Work on mobility and get physical activity on your rest days.

•Assess yourself after six weeks.

DAY 1: CHEST, BACK, ARMS

Warm-up: Pole assisted chest stretch, low squat semi-hang, biceps stretch, triceps stretch, forearm stretch, push-up.

Exercise	Set	Rep	
Bench Press	3	8 to 10	•Perform all sets in sequence with 1-3 minutes rest in between.
Barbell Row	3	8 to 10	•Work up to HEAVY WEIGHT for barbell bench press and barbell row.
Barbell Curl	3	10 to 12	•Use MEDIUM TO HEAVY WEIGHT for incline DB row and barbell curl.
Pull-up	3	5 to 8	•Subsitute dumbbells if barbell bench press causes shoulder pain.
Dip	3	10 to 15	•Always do an unloaded barbell set before adding weight to bench press.

DAY 2: LEGS, SHOULDERS (DEADLIFT CENTRIC)

Warm-up: Quadriceps stretch, hip flexors stretch, hamstrings stretch, pole assisted shoulder stretch, bodyweight squat.

Exercise	Set	Rep	
Split Squat	2	10 PER SIDE	•Perform all sets in sequence with 1-3 minutes rest in between.
Hip Bridge	2	15	•Work up to HEAVY WEIGHT for deadlift.
Deadlift	5	5	•Use LIGHT TO MEDIUM WEIGHT for barbell back lunge.
Barbell Back Lunge	5	10 PER SIDE	•Work up to HEAVY WEIGHT for OH barbell press.
OH Barbell Press	5	5 to 10	•Always do an unloaded barbell set before adding weight to barbell squat.

DAY 3: BACK, CHEST, ARMS, ABS (CALISTHENICS CENTRIC)
Warm-up: Pole assisted chest stretch, low squat semi-hang, push-up, bodyweight row.

Exercise	Set	Rep	
Pull-up	3	5 to 8	·Perform all sets in sequence with 1-3 minutes rest in between.
Single Bar Dip	3	10	·No free weights today.
Explosive Pull-up	3	3	
Push-up	3	15	
Hanging Leg Raise	3	10	

DAY 4: LEGS (SQUAT CENTRIC)
Warm-up: Quadriceps stretch, hip flexors stretch, hamstrings stretch, pole assisted shoulder stretch, bodyweight squat.

Exercise	Set	Rep	
Split Squat (PER SIDE)	3	10	·Perform all sets in sequence with 1-3 minutes rest in between.
Barbell Squat	4	10	·Work up to HEAVY WEIGHT for barbell squat.
One Leg Squat (SELF ASSISTED, PER SIDE)	3	1 to 3	·Always do an unloaded barbell set before adding weight to barbell squat.
Bulgarian Split Squat (PER SIDE)	3	10	

DAY 5: CHEST, BACK, SHOULDERS, ARMS, ABS (UPPER BODY PUSH/PULL)
Warm-up: Pole assisted chest stretch, low squat semi-hang, low abs stretch, biceps stretch, triceps stretch, forearm stretch, push-up.

Exercise	Set	Rep	
Bench Press	4	8 to 10	·This workout consists of several supersets of opposing muscle groups.
Pull-up	4	5 to 8	·Perform one set of bench press followed by one set of pull-ups. Repeat four times.
Handstand Push-up	4	1 to 2	·Perform one set of HSPU followed by one set of explosive pull-ups. Repeat four times.
Explosive Pull-up	4	1 to 3	·Perform one set of curls followed by one set of dips. Repeat four times.
DB Curl	4	10	·Perform one set of sit-ups followed by one set of hanging leg raises. Repeat four times.
Dip	3	10 to 15	·Use MEDIUM WEIGHT for barbell bench press and barbell row.
Sit-up	4	20	·Subsitute dumbbells if barbell bench press causes shoulder pain.
Hanging Leg Raise	4	10	·Always do an unloaded barbell set before adding weight to bench press.
			·If unable to do handstand push-ups then substitute MEDIUM to HEAVY overhead press.
			·Use MEDIUM to HEAVY weight for curls.

HELLYEAH! WEEK 2

DAY 1: CHEST, BACK, ARMS
Warm-up: Pole assisted chest stretch, low squat semi-hang, biceps stretch, triceps stretch, forearm stretch, push-up.

Exercise	Set	Rep
Bench Press	3	8 to 10
Barbell Row	3	8 to 10
Barbell Curl	3	10 to 12
Pull-up	3	5 to 8
Dip	3	10 to 15

·Perform all sets in sequence with 1-3 minutes rest in between.

·Work up to HEAVY WEIGHT for barbell bench press and barbell row.

·Use MEDIUM TO HEAVY WEIGHT for incline DB row and barbell curl.

·Subsitute dumbbells if barbell bench press causes shoulder pain.

·Always do an unloaded barbell set before adding weight to bench press.

DAY 2: LEGS, SHOULDERS (DEADLIFT CENTRIC)
Warm-up: Quadriceps stretch, hip flexors stretch, hamstrings stretch, pole assisted shoulder stretch, bodyweight squat.

Exercise	Set	Rep
Split Squat	2	10 PER SIDE
Hip Bridge	2	15
Deadlift	5	5
Barbell Back Lunge	5	10 PER SIDE
OH Barbell Press	5	5 to 10

·Perform all sets in sequence with 1-3 minutes rest in between.

·Work up to HEAVY WEIGHT for deadlift.

·Use LIGHT TO MEDIUM WEIGHT for barbell back lunge.

·Work up to HEAVY WEIGHT for OH barbell press.

·Always do an unloaded barbell set before adding weight to barbell squat.

DAY 3: BACK, CHEST, ARMS, ABS (CALISTHENICS CENTRIC)
Warm-up: Pole assisted chest stretch, low squat semi-hang, push-up, bodyweight row.

Exercise	Set	Rep
Pull-up	3	5 to 8
Single Bar Dip	3	10
Explosive Pull-up	3	3
Push-up	3	15
Hanging Leg Raise	3	10

·Perform all sets in sequence with 1-3 minutes rest in between.

·No free weights today.

DAY 4: LEGS (SQUAT CENTRIC)
Warm-up: Quadriceps stretch, hip flexors stretch, hamstrings stretch, pole assisted shoulder stretch, bodyweight squat.

Exercise	Set	Rep	
Split Squat (PER SIDE)	3	10	*•Perform all sets in sequence with 1-3 minutes rest in between.*
Barbell Squat	4	10	*•Work up to HEAVY WEIGHT for barbell squat.*
One Leg Squat (SELF ASSISTED, PER SIDE)	3	1 to 3	*•Always do an unloaded barbell set before adding weight to barbell squat.*
Bulgarian Split Squat (PER SIDE)	3	10	

DAY 5: CHEST, BACK, SHOULDERS, ARMS, ABS (UPPER BODY PUSH/PULL)
Warm-up: Pole assisted chest stretch, low squat semi-hang, low abs stretch, biceps stretch, triceps stretch, forearm stretch, push-up.

Exercise	Set	Rep	
Bench Press	4	8 to 10	*•This workout consists of several supersets of opposing muscle groups.*
Pull-up	4	5 to 8	*•Perform one set of bench press followed by one set of pull-ups. Repeat four times.*
Handstand Push-up	4	1 to 2	*•Perform one set of HSPU followed by one set of explosive pull-ups. Repeat four times.*
Explosive Pull-up	4	1 to 3	*•Perform one set of curls followed by one set of dips. Repeat four times.*
DB Curl	4	10	*•Perform one set of sit-ups followed by one set of hanging leg raises. Repeat four times.*
Dip	4	10 to 15	*•Use MEDIUM WEIGHT for barbell bench press and barbell row.*
Sit-up	4	20	*•Subsitute dumbbells if barbell bench press causes shoulder pain.*
Hanging Leg Raise	4	10	*•Always do an unloaded barbell set before adding weight to bench press.*
			•If unable to do handstand push-ups then substitute MEDIUM to HEAVY overhead press.
			•Use MEDIUM to HEAVY weight for curls.

HELLYEAH! *WEEK 3*

DAY 1: CHEST, BACK, ARMS
Warm-up: Pole assisted chest stretch, low squat semi-hang, biceps stretch, triceps stretch, forearm stretch, push-up.

Exercise	Set	Rep
Bench Press	3	8 to 10
Incine DB Press	3	10 to 12
Barbell Row	3	8 to 10
DB Row (PER ARM)	2	10
Barbell Curl	3	10 to 12
Pull-up	3	5 to 8
Dip	3	10 to 15

•Perform all sets in sequence with 1-3 minutes rest in between.

•Work up to HEAVY WEIGHT for barbell bench press and barbell row.

•Use MEDIUM TO HEAVY WEIGHT for incline DB press, DB row and barbell curl.

•Subsitute dumbbells if barbell bench press causes shoulder pain.

•Always do an unloaded barbell set before adding weight to bench press.

DAY 2: LEGS, SHOULDERS (DEADLIFT CENTRIC)
Warm-up: Quadriceps stretch, hip flexors stretch, hamstrings stretch, pole assisted shoulder stretch, bodyweight squat

Exercise	Set	Rep
Split Squat	2	10 PER SIDE
Weighted Split Squat	2	10 PER SIDE
Hip Bridge	2	15
Deadlift	5	5
Barbell Back Lunge	5	10 PER SIDE
OH Barbell Press	5	10

•Perform all sets in sequence with 1-3 minutes rest in between.

•Work up to HEAVY WEIGHT for deadlift.

•Use LIGHT TO MEDIUM WEIGHT for barbell back lunge.

•Work up to HEAVY WEIGHT for OH barbell press.

•Always do an unloaded barbell set before adding weight to barbell squat.

DAY 3: BACK, CHEST, ARMS, ABS (CALISTHENICS CENTRIC)
Warm-up: Pole assisted chest stretch, low squat semi-hang, push-up, bodyweight row.

Exercise	Set	Rep
Pull-up	3	8 to 10
Single Bar Dip	3	10
Explosive Pull-up	3	3
Muscle-up	3	1 to 3
Push-up	3	20
Hanging Leg Raise	3	15
Crossover Hanging Leg Raise	3	10

•Perform all sets in sequence with 1-3 minutes rest in between.

•This is a calisthenics based workout.

DAY 4: LEGS (SQUAT CENTRIC)
Warm-up: Quadriceps stretch, hip flexors stretch, hamstrings stretch, pole assisted shoulder stretch, bodyweight squat.

Exercise	Set	Rep
Split Squat (PER SIDE)	3	10
Weighted Split Squat (PER SIDE)	2	10
Barbell Squat	4	10
One Leg Squat (PER SIDE)	3	1 to 3
Bulgarian Split Squat (PER SIDE)	3	10

•Perform all sets in sequence with 1-3 minutes rest in between.

•Use MEDIUM WEIGHT for weighted split squat.

•Work up to HEAVY WEIGHT for barbell squat.

•Always do an unloaded barbell set before adding weight to barbell squat.

•If you are unable to perform a one leg squat, then continue to assist yourself.

DAY 5: CHEST, BACK, SHOULDERS, ARMS, ABS (UPPER BODY PUSH/PULL)
Warm-up: Pole assisted chest stretch, low squat semi-hang, low abs stretch, biceps stretch, triceps stretch, forearm stretch, push-up.

Exercise	Set	Rep
Bench Press	4	8 to 10
Pull-up	4	8 to 10
Handstand Push-up	4	2 to 3
Explosive Pull-up	4	1 to 4
DB Curl	4	10
Dip	4	10 to 15
Sit-up	4	30
Hanging Leg Raise	4	10

•This workout consists of several supersets of opposing muscle groups.

•Perform one set of bench press followed by one set of pull-ups. Repeat four times.

•Perform one set of HSPU followed by one set of explosive pull-ups. Repeat four times.

•Perform one set of curls followed by one set of dips. Repeat four times.

•Perform one set of sit-ups followed by one set of hanging leg raises. Repeat four times.

•Use MEDIUM WEIGHT for barbell bench press and barbell row.

•Subsitute dumbbells if barbell bench press causes shoulder pain.

•Always do an unloaded barbell set before adding weight to bench press.

•If unable to do handstand push-ups then substitute MEDIUM to HEAVY overhead press.

•Use MEDIUM to HEAVY weight for curls.

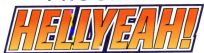

WEEK 4

DAY 1: CHEST, BACK, ARMS
Warm-up: Pole assisted chest stretch, low squat semi-hang, biceps stretch, triceps stretch, forearm stretch, push-up.

Exercise	Set	Rep
Bench Press	3	8 to 10
Incine DB Press	3	10 to 12
Barbell Row	3	8 to 10
DB Row (PER ARM)	2	10
Barbell Curl	3	10 to 12
Pull-up	3	5 to 8
Dip	3	10 to 15

·Perform all sets in sequence with 1-3 minutes rest in between.

·Work up to HEAVY WEIGHT for barbell bench press and barbell row.

·Use MEDIUM TO HEAVY WEIGHT for incline DB press, DB row and barbell curl.

·Subsitute dumbbells if barbell bench press causes shoulder pain.

·Always do an unloaded barbell set before adding weight to bench press.

DAY 2: LEGS, SHOULDERS (DEADLIFT CENTRIC)
Warm-up: Quadriceps stretch, hip flexors stretch, hamstrings stretch, pole assisted shoulder stretch, bodyweight squat.

Exercise	Set	Rep
Split Squat	2	10 PER SIDE
Weighted Split Squat	2	10 PER SIDE
Hip Bridge	2	15
Deadlift	5	5
Barbell Back Lunge	5	10 PER SIDE
OH Barbell Press	5	10

·Perform all sets in sequence with 1-3 minutes rest in between.

·Work up to HEAVY WEIGHT for deadlift.

·Use LIGHT TO MEDIUM WEIGHT for barbell back lunge.

·Work up to HEAVY WEIGHT for OH barbell press.

·Always do an unloaded barbell set before adding weight to barbell squat.

DAY 3: BACK, CHEST, ARMS, ABS (CALISTHENICS CENTRIC)
Warm-up: Pole assisted chest stretch, low squat semi-hang, push-up, bodyweight row.

Exercise	Set	Rep
Pull-up	3	8 to 10
Single Bar Dip	3	10
Explosive Pull-up	3	3
Muscle-up	3	1 to 3
Push-up	3	20
Hanging Leg Raise	3	15
Crossover Hanging Leg Raise	3	10

·Perform all sets in sequence with 1-3 minutes rest in between.

·This is a calisthenics based workout.

DAY 4: LEGS (SQUAT CENTRIC)
Warm-up: Quadriceps stretch, hip flexors stretch, hamstrings stretch, pole assisted shoulder stretch, bodyweight squat.

Exercise	Set	Rep	
Split Squat (PER SIDE)	3	10	*·Perform all sets in sequence with 1-3 minutes rest in between.*
Weighted Split Squat (PER SIDE)	2	10	*·Use MEDIUM WEIGHT for weighted split squat.*
Barbell Squat	4	10	*·Work up to HEAVY WEIGHT for barbell squat.*
One Leg Squat (PER SIDE)	3	1 to 3	*·Always do an unloaded barbell set before adding weight to barbell squat.*
Bulgarian Split Squat (PER SIDE)	3	10	*·If you are unable to perform a one leg squat, then continue to assist yourself.*

DAY 5: CHEST, BACK, SHOULDERS, ARMS, ABS (UPPER BODY PUSH/PULL)
Warm-up: Pole assisted chest stretch, low squat semi-hang, low abs stretch, biceps stretch, triceps stretch, forearm stretch, push-up.

Exercise	Set	Rep	
Bench Press	4	8 to 10	*·This workout consists of several supersets of opposing muscle groups.*
Pull-up	4	8 to 10	*·Perform one set of bench press followed by one set of pull-ups. Repeat four times.*
Handstand Push-up	4	2 to 3	*·Perform one set of HSPU followed by one set of explosive pull-ups. Repeat four times.*
Explosive Pull-up	4	1 to 4	*·Perform one set of curls followed by one set of dips. Repeat four times.*
DB Curl	4	10	*·Perform one set of sit-ups followed by one set of hanging leg raises. Repeat four times.*
Dip	4	10 to 15	*·Use MEDIUM WEIGHT for barbell bench press and barbell row.*
Sit-up	4	30	*·Subsitute dumbbells if barbell bench press causes shoulder pain.*
Hanging Leg Raise	4	10	*·Always do an unloaded barbell set before adding weight to bench press.*
			·If unable to do handstand push-ups then substitute MEDIUM to HEAVY overhead press.
			·Use MEDIUM to HEAVY weight for curls.

HELLYEAH! *WEEK 5*

DAY 1: CHEST, BACK, ARMS
Warm-up: Pole assisted chest stretch, low squat semi-hang, biceps stretch, triceps stretch, forearm stretch, push-up.

Exercise	Set	Rep	
Bench Press	3	8 to 10	•Perform all sets in sequence with 1-3 minutes rest in between.
Incine DB Press	3	10 to 12	•Work up to HEAVY WEIGHT for barbell bench press and barbell row.
DB Fly	3	15	•Work up to HEAVY WEIGHT for incline DB press, DB row and barbell curl.
Barbell Row	3	8 to 10	
DB Row (PER ARM)	2	10	•Subsitute dumbbells if barbell bench press causes shoulder pain.
Barbell Curl	3	10 to 12	•Use LIGHT WEIGHT for DB flys.
Pull-up	3	5 to 8	•Always do an unloaded barbell set before adding weight to bench press.
Dip	3	10 to 15	
Chin-up	2	MAX REPS	

DAY 2: LEGS, SHOULDERS (DEADLIFT CENTRIC)
Warm-up: Quadriceps stretch, hip flexors stretch, hamstrings stretch, pole assisted shoulder stretch, bodyweight squat.

Exercise	Set	Rep	
Split Squat	2	10 PER SIDE	•Perform all sets in sequence with 1-3 minutes rest in between.
Weighted Split Squat	2	10 PER SIDE	•Work up to HEAVY WEIGHT for deadlift.
Hip Bridge	2	15	•Use MEDIUM WEIGHT for weighted split squat and barbell back lunge.
Deadlift	5	5	•Work up to HEAVY WEIGHT for OH barbell press.
Barbell Back Lunge	5	10 PER SIDE	•Always do an unloaded barbell set before adding weight to barbell squat.
OH Barbell Press	5	10	

DAY 3: BACK, CHEST, ARMS, ABS (CALISTHENICS CENTRIC)
Warm-up: Pole assisted chest stretch, low squat semi-hang, push-up, bodyweight row.

Exercise	Set	Rep	
Pull-up	3	10	•Perform all sets in sequence with 1-3 minutes rest in between.
Single Bar Dip	3	10	•This is a calisthenics based workout.
Explosive Pull-up	3	1 to 5	
Muscle-up	3	1 to 5	
Push-up	3	25	
Hanging Leg Raise	3	20	
Crossover Hanging Leg Raise	3	15	

DAY 4: LEGS (SQUAT CENTRIC)

Warm-up: Quadriceps stretch, hip flexors stretch, hamstrings stretch, pole assisted shoulder stretch, bodyweight squat.

Exercise	Set	Rep	
Split Squat (PER SIDE)	3	10	•Perform all sets in sequence with 1-3 minutes rest in between.
Weighted Split Squat (PER SIDE)	2	10	•Use MEDIUM WEIGHT for weighted split squat.
Barbell Squat	4	10	•Work up to HEAVY WEIGHT for barbell squat.
One Leg Squat (PER SIDE)	3	2 to 3	•Always do an unloaded barbell set before adding weight to barbell squat.
Bulgarian Split Squat (PER SIDE)	3	10	•If you are unable to perform a one leg squat, then continue to assist yourself.

DAY 5: CHEST, BACK, SHOULDERS, ARMS, ABS (UPPER BODY PUSH/PULL)

Warm-up: Pole assisted chest stretch, low squat semi-hang, low abs stretch, biceps stretch, triceps stretch, forearm stretch, push-up.

Exercise	Set	Rep	
Bench Press	4	8 to 10	•This workout consists of several supersets of opposing muscle groups.
Pull-up	4	10+	•Perform one set of bench press followed by one set of pull-ups. Repeat four times.
Handstand Push-up	4	3 to 4	•Perform one set of HSPU followed by one set of explosive pull-ups. Repeat four times.
Explosive Pull-up	4	1 to 5	•Perform one set of curls followed by one set of dips. Repeat four times.
DB Curl	4	10	•Perform one set of sit-ups followed by one set of hanging leg raises. Repeat four times.
Dip	4	10 to 15	•Work up to HEAVY WEIGHT for barbell bench press and barbell row.
Sit-up	4	40	•Subsitute dumbbells if barbell bench press causes shoulder pain.
Hanging Leg Raise	4	10	•Always do an unloaded barbell set before adding weight to bench press.
			•If unable to do handstand push-ups then substitute MEDIUM to HEAVY overhead press.
			•Use MEDIUM to HEAVY weight for curls.

PROGRAM 3
HELLYEAH! WEEK 6

DAY 1: CHEST, BACK, ARMS
Warm-up: Pole assisted chest stretch, low squat semi-hang, biceps stretch, triceps stretch, forearm stretch, push-up.

Exercise	Set	Rep
Bench Press	3	8 to 10
Incine DB Press	3	10 to 12
DB Fly	3	15
Barbell Row	3	8 to 10
DB Row (PER ARM)	2	10
Barbell Curl	3	10 to 12
Pull-up	3	5 to 8
Dip	3	10 to 15
Chin-up	2	MAX REPS

- Perform all sets in sequence with 1-3 minutes rest in between.
- Work up to HEAVY WEIGHT for barbell bench press and barbell row.
- Work up to HEAVY WEIGHT for incline DB press, DB row and barbell curl.
- Subsitute dumbbells if barbell bench press causes shoulder pain.
- Use LIGHT WEIGHT for DB flys.
- Always do an unloaded barbell set before adding weight to bench press.

DAY 2: LEGS, SHOULDERS (DEADLIFT CENTRIC)
Warm-up: Quadriceps stretch, hip flexors stretch, hamstrings stretch, pole assisted shoulder stretch, bodyweight squat.

Exercise	Set	Rep
Split Squat	2	10 PER SIDE
Weighted Split Squat	2	10 PER SIDE
Hip Bridge	2	15
Deadlift	5	5
Barbell Back Lunge	5	10 PER SIDE
OH Barbell Press	5	10

- Perform all sets in sequence with 1-3 minutes rest in between.
- Work up to HEAVY WEIGHT for deadlift.
- Use MEDIUM WEIGHT for weighted split squat and barbell back lunge.
- Work up to HEAVY WEIGHT for OH barbell press.
- Always do an unloaded barbell set before adding weight to barbell squat.

DAY 3: BACK, CHEST, ARMS, ABS (CALISTHENICS CENTRIC)
Warm-up: Pole assisted chest stretch, low squat semi-hang, push-up, bodyweight row.

Exercise	Set	Rep
Pull-up	3	10
Single Bar Dip	3	10
Explosive Pull-up	3	1 to 5
Muscle-up	3	1 to 5
Push-up	3	25
Hanging Leg Raise	3	20
Crossover Hanging Leg Raise	3	15

- Perform all sets in sequence with 1-3 minutes rest in between.
- This is a calisthenics based workout.

DAY 4: LEGS (SQUAT CENTRIC)
Warm-up: Quadriceps stretch, hip flexors stretch, hamstrings stretch, pole assisted shoulder stretch, bodyweight squat.

Exercise	Set	Rep	
Split Squat (PER SIDE)	3	10	•Perform all sets in sequence with 1-3 minutes rest in between.
Weighted Split Squat (PER SIDE)	2	10	•Use MEDIUM WEIGHT for weighted split squat.
Barbell Squat	4	10	•Work up to HEAVY WEIGHT for barbell squat.
One Leg Squat (PER SIDE)	3	2 to 4	•Always do an unloaded barbell set before adding weight to barbell squat.
Bulgarian Split Squat (PER SIDE)	3	10	•If you are unable to perform a one leg squat, then continue to assist yourself.

DAY 5: CHEST, BACK, SHOULDERS, ARMS, ABS (UPPER BODY PUSH/PULL)
Warm-up: Pole assisted chest stretch, low squat semi-hang, low abs stretch, biceps stretch, triceps stretch, forearm stretch, push-up.

Exercise	Set	Rep	
Bench Press	4	8 to 10	•This workout consists of several supersets of opposing muscle groups.
Pull-up	4	10+	•Perform one set of bench press followed by one set of pull-ups. Repeat four times.
Handstand Push-up	4	3 to 4	•Perform one set of HSPU followed by one set of explosive pull-ups. Repeat four times.
Explosive Pull-up	4	1 to 5	•Perform one set of curls followed by one set of dips. Repeat four times.
DB Curl	4	10	•Perform one set of sit-ups followed by one set of hanging leg raises. Repeat four times.
Dip	4	10 to 15	•Work up to HEAVY WEIGHT for barbell bench press and barbell row.
Sit-up	4	40	•Subsitute dumbbells if barbell bench press causes shoulder pain.
Hanging Leg Raise	4	10	•Always do an unloaded barbell set before adding weight to bench press.
			•If unable to do handstand push-ups then substitute MEDIUM to HEAVY overhead press.
			•Use MEDIUM to HEAVY weight for curls.

PROGRAM 3

HELLYEAH!

ASSESS YOURSELF

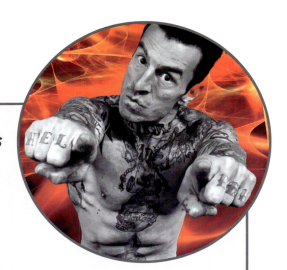

The following benchmarks serve as a measurable standard of achievement.

How do you measure up?

CAN YOU DO IT?

50 Push-ups	_____YES	_____NO
10 Pull-ups	_____YES	_____NO
1 Muscle-up	_____YES	_____NO
Squat 1.25x Bodyweight	_____YES	_____NO
Deadlift 2.25x Bodyweight	_____YES	_____NO

•*If YES TO ALL FIVE, then* HELLYEAH! *KEEP THE DREAM ALIVE!*

•*If NO, then repeat the last 2 weeks of* HELLYEAH!

•*If needed, add one day, specifically training the exercise(s) you did not complete in place of/in addition to Day 5.*

BONUS WORKOUTS

STEP UP YOUR SQUAT

The squat is one of the most important lifts there is. Here's how to get better at it. This program is based on volume and repetition. Use a spotter for heavy weight.

STEP UP YOUR SQUAT Warm-up: Quadriceps stretch, hip flexors stretch, hamstrings stretch, hands behind back stretch.			
Exercise	**Set**	**Rep**	·Perform the first three exercises in sequence with 1-2 minutes rest in between.
Bodyweight Squat	2	10	·You may take longer rest longer in between barbell squat sets.
Goblet Squat	3	10	·Use LIGHT WEIGHT for first set of barbell squats.
Bodyweight Split Squat (PER SIDE)	3	10	·Use MEDIUM WEIGHT for next 2-3 sets of barbell squats.
Barbell Squat	10	5	·Use HEAVY WEIGHT for remaining sets of barbell squats.
			·Do one LIGHT WEIGHT cool down set of barbell squats at the end of the workout.

MUSCLE MANIA

This is an advanced calisthenics upper body workout specifically designed to help you get better at muscle-ups. Although it is composed of tough exercises, this workout goes by quickly.

MUSCLE MANIA Warm-up: Bar hang, crescent moon, forearm stretch.			
Exercise	**Set**	**Rep**	·Perform the first three exercises in sequence with 1-2 minutes rest in between.
Pull-up	2	5 to 10	·You may take longer rest periods between explosive pull-ups and muscle-ups.
Single Bar Dip	3	5 to 10	*You may break the reps down into more sets if needed.
Explosive Pull-up	3	3 to 5	
Muscle-up	3 to 5	1 to 5	
Single Bar Dip	3	5	
Pull-up	2	5	

DEADLIFT DEATHSTROKE

Incorporating deadlifting in your program is one of the best ways to develop full body strength and power. I encourage you to go heavy, but do not sacrifice form. If form is compromised, then reduce the weight. Quality of movement is more important than quantity of weight.

DEADLIFT DEATHSTROKE Warm-up: Quadriceps stretch, hip flexors stretch, hamstrings stretch, forward bend.			
Exercise	**Set**	**Rep**	·Perform first three exercises in sequence with 1-2 minutes rest in between.
Bodyweight Squat	2	10	·You may take longer rest longer in between deadlift sets.
Bodyweight Split Squat (PER SIDE)	2	10	·Gradually increase weight for first three sets of deadlift to get fired up.
Hip Bridge	2	10	
Deadlift	3	5 to 8	·Use HEAVY WEIGHT for deadlift Round 2. Take longer rest periods if needed.
Deadlift (ROUND 2)	5	3 to 5	·You may substitue a trap bar for deadlift Round 2.
			·Do one LIGHT WEIGHT cool down set of deadlifts at the end of the workout.

DIAMOND-CUT ABS

Strength and health are two of the main benefits of training. Improved appearance is another. Forge the ultimate set of indestructible abdominals with this workout.

DIAMOND-CUT ABS Warm-up: Low abs stretch, seated twist, baby cobra.			
Exercise	**Set**	**Rep**	·Perform first three exercises in a circuit. Repeat three times.
Straight Leg Raise	3	25	·Perform last two exercises as supersets. Repeat two times.
Sit-up	3	25	·Substitute crossover hanging knee raise if crossover hanging leg raise is too difficult.
Crossover Sit-up (PER SIDE)	3	25	
Jackknife	2	25	
Crossover Hanging Leg Raise (PER SIDE)	2	10	

FLEX FACTOR

Flexibility training is just as vital and important as strength training. This is a series of forward, back and side bending stretches that targets every muscle group in your body.

<table>
<tr><td colspan="4">FLEX FACTOR
Warm-up: Sit still and breathe.</td></tr>
<tr><td>Exercise</td><td>Set</td><td>Rep</td><td>•Perform each stretch one time for 60 seconds.</td></tr>
<tr><td>Hands Behind Back</td><td></td><td></td><td rowspan="2">•Use the first 30 seconds to gradually push into your deepest hold.</td></tr>
<tr><td>Chest Stretch</td><td>2</td><td>60, 30 sec. hold</td></tr>
<tr><td>Crescent Moon</td><td>2</td><td>60, 30 sec. hold</td><td>•Use the second 30 seconds to hold this position.</td></tr>
<tr><td>Forward Bend</td><td>2</td><td>60, 30 sec. hold</td><td>•Take a few breaths after completing each stretch once.</td></tr>
<tr><td>Baby Cobra</td><td>2</td><td>60, 30 sec. hold</td><td rowspan="2">•For the second set, get into your deepest hold quickly and hold for 30 seconds.</td></tr>
<tr><td>Camel</td><td>2</td><td>60, 30 sec. hold</td></tr>
<tr><td>Seated Twist (PER SIDE)</td><td>2</td><td>60, 30 sec. hold</td><td></td></tr>
</table>

MORE ABOUT PROGRAMMING

FREQUENCY & RECOVERY

This refers to how often you train in a given time period (usually a week) and how many days you rest between training sessions. I recommend working out at least three days a week in order to get results. If you train more frequently, it is generally a good idea to "split" your workouts.

Full body workouts, where everything is targeted in the same session, cannot effectively be done more than three times a week; there's just not enough time to recover. That is why many prescribe a split exercise routine. This means that you train different body parts or muscle groups on different days so you can hit them harder, yet still give yourself enough recovery time between workouts. In other words, if you destroy your legs on Monday, then your next workout should target another muscle group or groups. Your exercise selection and workout intensity have to correspond to the frequency at which you train.

SEQUENCING

For the most part, a workout should start with a brief warm-up. The point of the warm-up is to prepare you mentally and physically. A warm-up can consist of stretching, mild cardio, mobility drills and/or light strength training.

Your warm-up is usually followed by one or more medium intensity exercises, after which comes the larger moves. These are either the heaviest lifts, most challenging skills or exercises that recruit the most muscle, such as squats, deadlifts, muscle-ups, handstand push-ups, heavy presses, etc. It's important to work on these exercises somewhat early in the workout while your energy levels are still high, but not so soon that you're unprepared. Perform the smaller, supplemental exercises after the larger, power moves.

This is a general template on which to base your workouts. Naturally, there are others as well. The most important aspect of any exercise sequence is that the practitioner is focused, hard-working and committed.

ACTIVE RECOVERY

Active recovery is another type of exercise sequencing. Most of the time, you rest in between sets and exercises. Perform one set, rest then repeat. Active recovery means that instead of resting, you do a different exercise that focuses on another body part or muscle group, while the first one recovers. This allows you to get more done in less time and also provides a peripheral conditioning effect. "Supersets", where you do two exercises back to back before resting (see Program 3, Day 5) and "circuit training", where you perform a whole series of exercises with little or no rest in between (see Program 1, Day 3) are both examples of active recovery.

SETS & REPS

There is an infinite number of set and rep schemes, and to be candid, they are all more effective than not having a plan at all. Over the course of time, however, some set and rep schemes have gained particular favor for producing targeted results. Here is the breakdown:

3x10 This is probably the most popular set/rep combo in all of strength training. What's not to love? We have ten fingers, ten toes and a base-ten numeral system. We love the *Three Musketeers, the Three Little Pigs* and even *the Three Stooges!* There's a human fondness of these numbers. But the real reason more kids start out lifting weights in this template is because it works! For best results, use a weight or choose an exercise where the last few reps are very tough—they're the ones that count. If ten reps comes easy, then you need to add more weight or do a harder exercise.

3x12 to 15 This combination works along the same principle as 3x10. The idea here is to wear the muscle down by replacing some of the resistance with volume. Generally, I like doing 3x15 with exercises that train smaller muscles or bend at shallow joints (curls, lateral raises, flys, etc.) For the most part, size and strength are built in the 8-15 rep range.

5x10, 10x10 Sometimes more is more. Think of this as the classic 3x10, but more. Possibly much more. Increasing the number of sets is a simple and time tested way of achieving greater volume in one workout. This template will help you grow stronger and more proficient at almost any exercise. Allow plenty of time for your workouts. In addition to the added volume, you'll need more recovery time between sets.

5x5, 5x3, 10x5, 6x2, etc. This template is also along the "more is more" concept. Doing fewer reps per set allows you to go heavier. Use this template when you desire multiple repetitions of maximum force. To be most effective, the exercise must be extremely challenging in the low rep range. I generally program 5x5 or 5x3 for heavy deadlifts, muscle-ups and one leg squats. Make sure you are warmed up and take appropriate recovery time between sets.

High Repetition (25+) After about 25 reps of many strength exercises, if you're able to keep going, then it becomes more about muscular endurance than strength. For example, there comes a point where all the bodyweight squats in the world will cease to build muscle. That is when it's time to do a more advanced bodyweight exercise, add resistance or both. Pull-up variations, by contrast, do not fall into this category as the genetic potential to perform a large number within a single set is limited. In fact, the ability to perform just one set of twenty pull-ups is rare, even within fitness circles, so feel free to max out on your pull-ups. Not all exercises have the same demand.

HITTING A MAX

Tracking your maximum efforts is a helpful tool for assessing your progress. For calisthenics exercises like push-ups, pull-ups and muscle-ups, "hitting a max" usually refers to your *max reps*, or the highest number of repetitions you can perform in one single, unbroken set. For weight training exercises like squats, deadlifts and bench press, the phrase signifies your *one rep max*, or the greatest external weight you can wield for one repetition. In either case, in order for a max effort to count, you must use proper form.

I'd like to be clear that when I discuss training for a one rep max, it's solely for the sake of tracking your results, <u>NOT</u> training for a competition. Competitive powerlifting and Olympic weightlifting are specific pursuits with their own protocol. Still, whether you're an Olympian or not, performing a true max means that you put forth your greatest effort. I don't recommend attempting a max lift more than about once every three months. Some coaches recommend no more than twice a year.

Like most aspects of fitness, there is no single, one-size-fits-all approach to hitting a max lift. Individuals will need to experiment. Here are some guidelines:

- You need to be at your peak. If you're feeling sub-par, save it for another day.

- Start out with a warm-up consisting of mobility and dynamic movement.

- Perform 1 to 3 light to medium weight sets.

- When you're physically and mentally primed, perform sets of 1-3 reps, increasing the load in increments of approximately 10-20% of your current max. If you don't know your max, then err on the side of caution.

- When you're close to your current one rep max, perform 1 rep at a time and increase the load in smaller increments.

- You will need longer rest periods than usual between sets.

Working towards a max in calisthenics calls for a different approach. Since you can't change what your body weighs between sets, we do max reps. This can be done far more frequently than training for a one rep max in weight lifting. Here are two approaches:

1. Muscular Failure Method - To perform maximum repetitions of any exercise, you need to get conditioned to volume and discomfort. Therefore, I recommend adding at least two sets to complete failure. If you want to increase your dips, for example, then add two sets to failure early in your workout on your regular dip day. You may also add a third "burnout" set at the end of the workout.

2. "Get In When You Fit In" Method - Targeting the goal exercise on a non-training day is another favorable approach. Since you're essentially adding some strength work to what was a non-strength day, think of this as "practicing" rather than exercising. Instead of a formal workout, simply do a few sets throughout the day with lots of time in between. These sets should be about half your current max. In other words, if you can do 8 unbroken pull-ups at your best, then do several sets of 4. Take anywhere from 30 minutes to two hours in between.

Maxing out on weighted calisthenics calls for a similar approach to weight training. We test for one rep max. In fact, one could truthfully argue that a barbell squat is weighted calisthenics, so why should we train a weighted one leg squat (or pull-up or dip) much differently?

Attempting a weighted calisthenics max is not an exact science, but there are several guidelines to consider. Here they are:

- Weighted pull-ups, dips and one leg squats can place an unexpected amount of stress on your joints and connective tissue. While healthy joints can handle it, it's still best to progress slowly.

- Start out with a warm-up consisting of mobility and dynamic movement.

- Perform 1 to 2 unweighted sets.

- When you're physically and mentally primed, perform a weighted set of 1-3 reps, at approximately 25% of your current max. Increase the load in increments of approximately 25-30% of your current max. If you don't know your max, then err on the side of caution.

- When you're close to your current max, perform 1 rep at a time, increasing the load in smaller increments.

- You will need longer rest periods than usual between sets.

SCHEDULING

Scheduling is key for accountability. If you don't make time for your workouts, they will not happen. That said, depending on your work schedule, family life and other commitments, what time of day you work out may be dictated more by necessity than preference. Of course, if you have the opportunity to train when it's optimal for you, then go for it. I personally do my workouts as early in the day as my schedule permits, but I've known others who prefer afternoons or evenings.

As for which days to train, once again, outside circumstances come into play. But in almost every situation, it's best to hit it hard on Monday and not take off early in the week. Time has a way of going by quickly and it's helpful to get a jump start. If you front load your week with hard work, there's less chance of missing a workout.

Still, unexpected things can happen, and if you do miss a workout, don't become derailed. Forgive yourself and prioritize the next one. Working out requires commitment and follow-through. In order to be consistent, you must allocate the time.

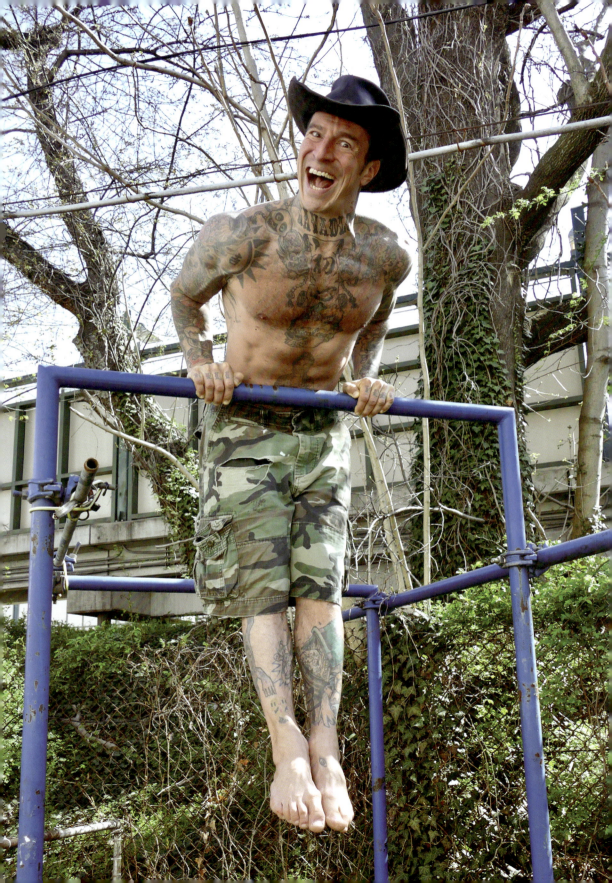

PART V

MOVING FORWARD

As we continue our training over the years (*you don't stop just because you completed a program*), it's important to remain open to new feedback. Pay attention to first hand experience. Oftentimes, it's the best teacher.

At the same time, try to avoid falling into an unquestioning mindset. It's a mistake to think we know it all. When we stop asking questions, we stop getting answers. The man who claims to completely know himself is selling himself short.

One should never be afraid to learn, grow and gain further insight. Moving forward in fitness, there is always more to consider.

Our lifestyle choices affect everything we do, not just our training. The decisions we make outside the gym have a greater impact than even the exercise itself.

I hope you revisit these pages in the forthcoming months and years, as we continue to grow strong and amazing together.

FREQUENTLY ASKED QUESTIONS

Q: I just started working out and my muscles are getting sore. Is that bad?

A: *Probably not. In fact, some degree of muscular soreness, particularly if you're a beginner or haven't worked out in a while, is a good sign that your muscles are working hard. The soreness is a byproduct of strength training. The muscle has to get damaged in order to repair and grow. That's what you're feeling.*

Q: I've been working out for a while and my muscles are no longer getting sore. Is that bad?

A: *Probably not. It means that your muscles are adapting to exercise. The amount of muscular soreness one experiences from a workout is not the greatest indicator of the quality of said workout. Much of the time, muscles get sore when they are put to a new task. Therefore, as you get better at any particular exercise, it becomes less shocking to your system and doesn't make you as sore as it used to. We need to continually challenge ourselves if we want to make gains, but after working out for years, you may never feel as sore as you did at the beginning, even when training really, really hard.*

Q: What about overtraining?

A: *Overtraining can be a real concern, just not for the average guy or gal who works out, even most fitness fanatics. For most people, undertraining is a more realistic concern. The body can take a lot and many of us could probably afford to step up our workouts, if anything. Yes, there are competitive athletes who train excruciatingly long sessions in extreme conditions, and they may run the possible risk of overtraining. Until the day comes when you and I find ourselves in a similar situation, we need not be too concerned. Don't confuse working hard with overtraining.*

Q: I need to lose weight by this summer. What is the best exercise for weight loss?

A: *Simply eating less (and better) food will have a greater impact than all the exercise in the world. In order to lose weight you will need to burn more fuel than you are putting in. Doing so causes your body to metabolize stored glycogen and, ultimately, fat. You need to go without in order to lose weight. If you're eating every few hours, your body never has a cause to burn fat. While nutrition is far more nuanced than that, a caloric deficit is necessary for weight loss. Naturally, the quality of the food, as well as other factors, matter too.*

I've said many times that the food we choose to eat is the single biggest decision we can make regarding our fitness; this is true not only for overall health, but also specifically for weight loss. Take a look at the next chapter for all the nutritional guidance you'll need.

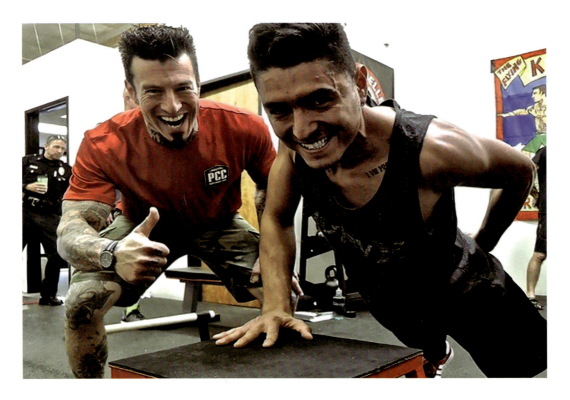

Q: I want to put on ten pounds of lean muscle in one month. Is that realistic?

A: *No, it's not. Your body needs time to manifest change and it's impossible to naturally synthesize that much lean mass so quickly. Think back to a time in your life when you've gained weight, lost weight or physically changed in any capacity at all. Chances are it was over the course of several weeks, months or even longer. Building muscle is a process that takes consistent effort over the course of years. The fact that there are no shortcuts is part of what gives it value. If it was quick or easy, then everyone would be huge. Clearly, that is not the case.*

For that matter, fitness deadlines in general are often thrown around a bit too liberally. ("I'm gonna bench 315 this summer"; "I'm learning a muscle-up this week"; "I'm doing fifty pull-ups for my 50th birthday!") And while there's no doubt that deadlines can have value, they can also instill unrealistic expectations and disappointment. It's good to look into the future but we must live in the present.

Q: How should I breathe during exercise?

A: *I do not have one general, blanket rule when it comes to breathing. In much of strength training, we are taught to exhale for the concentric phase of an exercise and inhale for the eccentric phase. This is a good rule of thumb but it does not always apply.*

Sometimes it feels good to hold your breath, brace your belly and fill yourself with air in order to build tension. (This is sometimes referred to as the Valsalva maneuver.) Other times, you may prefer to breathe slowly and deeply in and out through your nostrils. Your breathing may even change from exercise to exercise... just don't forget to do it!

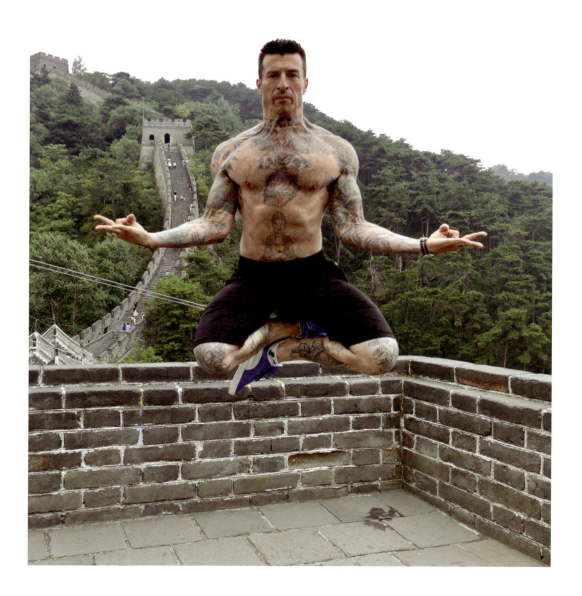

Q: Can I use gymnastic rings for pull-ups?

A: *Sure. Rings are a fine substitute if no bar is available. They work for bodyweight curls and rows as well. Additionally, since rings and other suspension trainers are not fixed, your arms can rotate at the shoulder joints during the exercise.*

Q: Why doesn't this book include decline bench press/one arm pull-up/snatch/box jump/etc.?

A: *No program can include everything. This is not to say that these non-included exercises do not have value — lots of things do. But the exercises included in this book are the ones I feel are most effective in general. That's why they're the ones I most often use for myself and my personal training clients.*

Q: Can teenagers lift weights?

A: *YES! Not only can teenagers lift weights — they should! I remember when I started lifting in the 1980's, there were all kinds of tales about how exercise stunts your growth. Though this absurd notion has been proven false time and time again, some parents still believe it (probably the parents who don't work out).*

The truth is that teenagers reap the same healthy, functional and aesthetic benefits as adults do from strength training, and they're even less prone to injury. Additionally, the changes that teenagers' bodies are already going through puts them at a great advantage in terms of muscle synthesis and recovery.

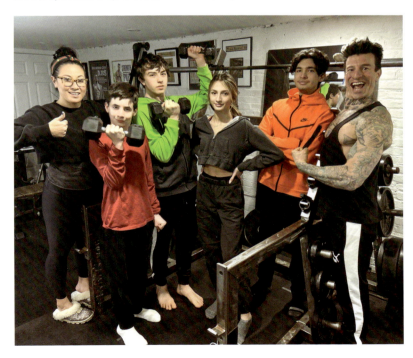

I've been running "Friday Fit Club" out of my basement gym since 2017. "FFC" is an opportunity for the neighborhood kids to train with me. It's also 100% free. Not only can teenagers lift weights — they should!

DANNY'S DOS AND DON'TS
NUTRITION & LIFESTYLE EDITION

DO TREAT PROBLEMS, NOT JUST SYMPTOMS

"We have made ourselves living cesspools, and driven doctors to invent names for our diseases." These words were written by Plato over 2,000 years ago and are still shockingly true today. We are so focused on sickness yet spend little time on wellness.

The cure for ailments ranging from heart disease to diabetes, acne to allergies, even depression and violence, is found in our diet, nutrition and lifestyle. As a culture we tend to treat symptoms, but not problems. The cause remains. For example, when an obese person's doctor prescribes cholesterol meds, it doesn't help the patient. In fact, it does the opposite. By enabling him or her to continue on a path toward self destruction, the physician discourages the patient from actually improving their health. Getting rid of the cause of high cholesterol is the answer, not masking the body's reaction to the problem.

This is not an indictment of medicine. Far from it. Homeopathic remedies are also deployed under the same guise. Whether you swallow a handful of pills peddled by a physician or drink a garlic/cayenne pepper juice sold by a hippie, you're treating inflammation, but not the reason for it. Symptoms, not problems. What are you putting in your body the rest of the time that caused this? It starts with daily habits.

The way to strengthen your systems is by eating lots of raw vegetables and fruits, exercising daily and exposing yourself to outdoor elements. If you pump yourself full of fake food, artificial preservatives and mind-altering (prescription and non-prescription) drugs on a regular basis, you don't stand a chance.

The toxic stuff we put in our body is the root of our unwellness. It is only through taking better care of ourselves that we can truly heal. I'll show you how. Keep reading.

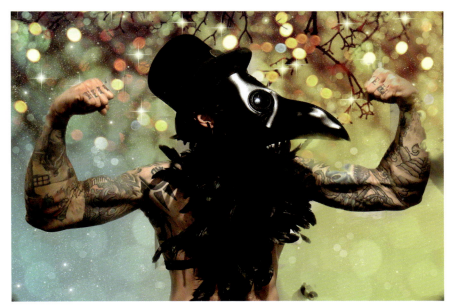

The doctor is in.

DO EAT SIMPLY

Because personal chemistry and environmental factors are different for everybody, the fine details of what's best to eat varies from person to person. It helps to do some personal experimentation. That said, some blanket concepts are universal. For starters, keep it simple.

I recommend eating mainly plants and animals, in that order. By plants, I mean lots of greens, beans, seeds, herbs, fruits and roots. These foods are loaded with nutrients and fiber. I suggest eating at least one giant, raw vegetable salad a day, and as many raw fruits and veggies as you want all day. Just remember, a green salad means veggies only—no bacon, chicken strips, blobs of cheese or ranch dressing. Instead, use lemon juice, vinegar with cracked pepper or nothing at all.

Let's also set the record straight about fruit, which sometimes gets a bum rap due to sugar content. Yes, although fruit contains natural, unprocessed sugar, it is loaded with fiber (not to mention vitamins, minerals and enzymes). Fruit is metabolized and absorbed slowly. Eating fruit is not the same as eating refined sugar, raw sugar or even honey. Plus fruit is naturally sweet and filling. Bring more fruit into your life and your candy cravings will plummet.

FIBER

Fiber (aka roughage or bulk) is non-digestible plant parts that help you maintain metabolic health, control your sugar levels and lower your cholesterol. Proteins, fats, vitamins and minerals are digested and absorbed. Since fiber is not, it helps carry waste from your body, and is important for bowel health (which is key to overall health). Fruits, vegetables, beans, nuts and grains are rich in fiber. Fiber should be eaten in just about every meal.

We also need protein for building muscle and repairing organs. Just not as much as we're often told. Humans are omnivores who thrive on a mostly vegetarian diet, supplemented with meat (beef, lamb, fowl, fish) and other animal proteins (eggs, yogurt, milk). While fruits and veggies can be consumed all day, every day, I recommend far fewer servings of animal protein, about five to fifteen per week. To be clear, a serving is the size of your palm, not your arm.

If you choose not to eat animals, other complete protein sources are available. These include nuts, legumes, seeds, mushrooms and certain greens. Just be aware that you'll have to eat a lot in order to match the quantity of protein in meat and dairy. For example, 100 grams of broccoli or spinach has about 2.5g of protein. The same weight of steak, chicken or fish has 25g or more — ten times as much!

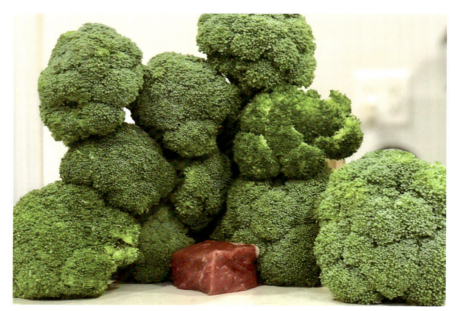

It would take a lot of broccoli to match the protein contained in a petite filet mignon, the smallest steakhouse cut.

I keep my consumption of grain products and sweets to a minimum. Usually when I say this, detractors will point out that eliminating carbohydrates is not a good long-term plan, as carbs are an effective source of energy... and they're right! That's why my main dietary recommendations (vegetables and fruits) are carbs. Corn, parsnips, potatoes and rutabagas are starchy carbs. We sometimes associate the word "carbohydrates" exclusively with grain products like bread, rice and pasta. For clarity, when I say to go lightly on grains and sweets, I don't mean all carbohydrates. I do not advocate the complete elimination of any macro-nutrients (proteins, fats, carbohydrates) or complete food group (meat, plants, bread, etc.)

Overly restrictive diets, especially those that vilify entire food groups, can lead to an abusive relationship with food. We never want that. Food is our friend, not just our fuel. That's part of what makes cooking is so special: not only do you know exactly what you're eating, but you also get to create it! There is a common misconception that those who choose to maintain a healthy weight do not enjoy food. Quite the contrary; most enjoy it more. We appreciate it because we're not desensitized to it.

When you eat simple, healthy and delicious foods most of the time, it's okay to enjoy an occasional, well deserved indulgence. A slice of cake is fine on your birthday — just not every day... and not the whole cake!

DO PRACTICE MINDFUL SHOPPING

When shopping, I stick to simple foods like produce, meats cut fresh from the butcher counter and breads baked close to home. As a general rule, we want to avoid overly processed, packaged foods. While it's worth noting that almost everything we eat is processed to some degree, not all processing is the same. For example, turning peanuts into peanut butter or spinach into spinach juice (both of which are technically "processed") are quite different from what's happening with a frozen chicken chimichanga.

If you do buy packaged foods, then read the list of ingredients. If you couldn't identify most of these ingredients if you saw them in person, then they probably are not food. Be sure to check on the "serving size" and "serving quantity" per package as well. Oftentimes, products that look like a single serving are considered to be many more by the manufacturer. If a box says three servings are contained, then multiply the calories, fat and sugar content on the label by three. Anything you don't use for energy will be converted to fat.

DO GET PHYSICAL AND MENTAL EXERCISE EVERY DAY

That's right. Every single day. To clarify, I don't mean that you need to lift weights seven days a week (although when done correctly, you may). Activities such as cycling, stretching, yoga and power walking are all forms of physical exercise. By incorporating them on your non-strength training days, you will remain spry and energized.

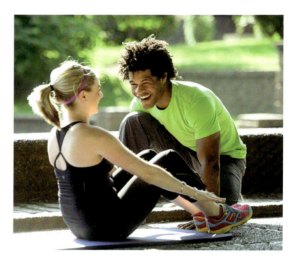

On the same note, we also need mental exercise. When we learn new information or a new skill, we stimulate the brain's activity and increase blood flow to the frontal cortex. It keeps us sharp. This does not happen when we revisit things we already knew. It's imperative that we challenge the mind, not just the body, with NEW information, skills and stimuli.

DO DRINK LOTS OF WATER AND LESS OF EVERYTHING ELSE

This may be trickier than it seems, as "everything else" does not just refer to sugary sodas and adult libations. It's common knowledge that they stand in the way of becoming jacked and shredded.

What may not be known is that vitamin water, sweetened coconut juices and coffee-inspired dessert beverages, while sometimes healthful looking, are also trash. Same for jacked up energy drinks, sports drinks and diet soda. Replace them all with good old H2O. If you drink coffee (black only, please) or tea (plain or with lemon) in the morning, then have a glass of water first.

Here are some of the benefits of drinking lots of water:

- Improved metabolic rate
- Better digestion
- Hydrated, moisturized skin
- Faster removal of toxins
- Better physical performance
- Higher energy levels
- Improved brain and organ function
- Bigger muscles

DON'T EAT SO MUCH SALT, SUGAR & FAT

It is in our animal nature to crave salt, sugar and fat. As hunter-gatherers living off the land, early humans needed salt for water retention, sugar for quick fuel and fat for warmth and stored energy. It was unknown when or where the next meal would come from, so we evolved to instinctively desire these hard to find foodstuffs for survival.

Fast forward to the 21st Century where we are surrounded by salt, sugar and fat at every turn. There is no scarcity, only a gross abundance. We therefore have to actively fight these cravings. Many Americans start the day with a sugary coffee concoction, then eat dessert for breakfast: chocolate muffins, frosty pink donuts and bagels with sweetened cream cheese. That's all before 9am and it's downhill from there. It's no wonder there is an obesity epidemic.

Food manufacturers and restaurants use salt, sugar and fat as culinary cheap thrills in order to appeal to our cravings. Too much of this leaves us flaccid, diseased and weak. Unfortunately, this practice is not limited to fast food burgers and gas station fried chicken. Most restaurants, including many that claim to be healthy, are drowning your food in cream, sweeteners and sodium behind closed doors. Much of the packaged food items sold in big supermarkets and chain stores is loaded with low quality incarnations of these substances as well. Cutting down on these components will leave you feeling stronger, leaner and more energized. Your food will taste better.

DON'T STAY UP SO LATE

The fitness industry places a tremendous amount of focus on exercise and diet. Sleep, though less of a hot topic, deserves an equal share of the spotlight.

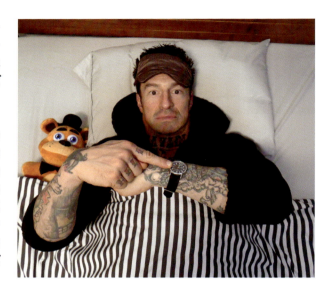

While individual sleep needs vary, it's safe to say that most adults require at least six or seven hours average per night in order to be dynamic and happy. Some need eight or more. Regardless of your specific sleep demands, none of us should underestimate the value of sleep, rest and recovery.

When you sleep, your organ tissues repair and rebuild. You are rewarded for all the work you did in the gym. (Remember, muscles grow when you recover NOT when you train.) Your hormones replenish and brain levels adjust. You simply feel better when you get ample rest.

Just like we have to allocate time for exercise, we need to delegate time for sleep. Anyone who wants to be more productive should turn off their phone and go to bed an hour earlier.

DON'T DRINK SO MUCH BOOZE AND SMOKE SO MUCH WEED

I know what you're thinking and yes, I like to party as much as the next guy — probably a lot more. And yes, I'm aware that a lot of jacked guys do, in fact, drink and smoke. I fully acknowledge that it is possible to be in shape if you drink alcohol or smoke marijuana — you're just making it much more difficult than it needs to be!

That stuff will hinder your gains.

I am not some teetotaler coming at this from a finger-wagging standpoint. I have nothing against catching a buzz. Grown-ups get to make their own decisions and I don't judge. However, if you want to get in peak shape, be aware that drinking too much alcohol will dehydrate you, impair your sleep and make it harder to synthesize muscle. Smoking anything will harm your respiratory system and interfere with oxygen and nutrient flow to the muscles you just trained. And while I've been known to indulge myself, I'll be the first to tell you: *marijuana will zap your workout intensity*. This temporary decline in mojo makes it harder for you to start and/or continue a tough workout. Although we love hearing good news about our bad habits, it's important to be realistic.

Sure, if you really want to enjoy a drink or a puff, then go for it. Just remember, it's a fine line between a little harmless recreation and something that holds you back.

DON'T LET TOXIC PEOPLE IN

Detox isn't always about food and drink. Toxic stressors are all around and can come in many forms, even as people. If you have folks in your life that consistently bring you pain, difficulty or grief, then you may have to reevaluate your choices. Engaging unnecessarily with fake friends or aggressive acquaintances only slows us down.

Of course, even our loved ones can get on our nerves at times. Indeed, we sometimes butt heads with people who are positive forces. That is not what I'm referring to. I'm talking about those who you've kept around in spite of a deteriorating, even harmful relationship: people you genuinely feel bad around. They are nothing more than time bandits, seeking to rob you of your most valued commodity. Don't take the bait. It's an exercise in futility and frustration.

DON'T WAIT FOR MOTIVATION

Motivation is great, but we can't wait for it to strike. You must put forth the effort, even when you don't feel like it. *Especially* when you don't feel like it.

If you're not getting the physique you desire, then ask yourself real questions and give truthful answers. Are you showing up? Are you missing too many workouts? Are you ready to work hard? Don't kid yourself. You'll need to make changes in your schedule and your efforts if you're serious about getting in shape. Anyone can work out when motivation strikes. Champions work out when it doesn't.

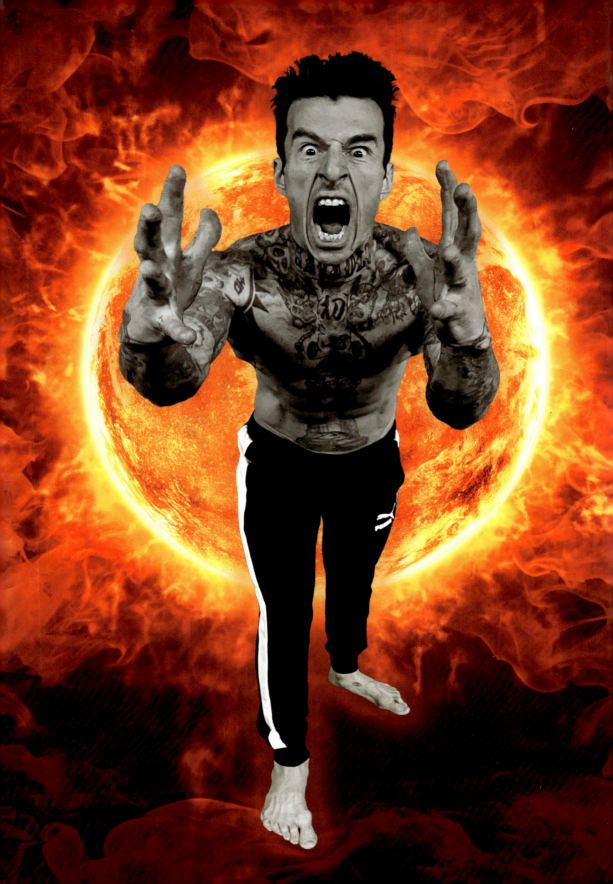

WALKING THROUGH FIRE

Human biology has not changed in hundreds of thousands of years. We're still creatures who need to move, run and climb, living in the land of Uber Eats and never-ending Zoom calls. The world around us is different, but our bodies are not. The struggle for existence is real.

It's alarming to ponder modern man's exaggerated waistline, hunched posture and inability to tolerate discomfort. Kids are growing up weaker and dumber than their parents. Life has gotten a little too easy. By contrast, we need difficulty to get stronger.

Poet Charles Bukowski wrote, "What matters most is how well you walk through the fire." Well, we are all walking through fire on this path toward health and strength. We need to move forward in spite of obstacles, whether real or perceived, to reach our goals, without fear of failure. The most successful people in the gym (and the world) have failed again and again in pursuit of success. When we are challenged — even when we lose — we are greater for it. No excuses.

Exercise challenges us in necessary ways. This concept is simple, though working out is not easy.

Life, however, is neither simple nor easy. It's complicated and nuanced. The one thing in this world that you have true control over is your own body, so take ownership!

Be strong, my friends. Walk through fire.

Keep the Dream alive!

ABOUT THE AUTHOR

Danny Kavadlo was born in Brooklyn, NY, eats mainly plants and animals and exercises every day Danny helped pioneer the bodyweight fitness craze with **Strength Rules**, **Diamond-Cut Abs** and **Get Strong**, all of which went to #1 on Amazon. He has been featured in the *New York Times, Huffington Post* and *Men's Health,* and is a contributor to *TRAIN* magazine and *Bodybuilding.com.* When he's not traveling the world as Master Instructor for Dragon Door's acclaimed PCC Certification, Danny works with personal training clients in New York City and virtual clients everywhere.

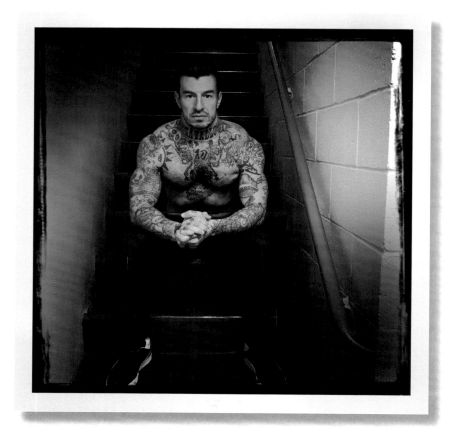

Find out more about Danny:
Instagram: @dannykavadlo
Facebook: www.facebook.com/DannyTheTrainer
Website: www.DannyTheTrainer.com

ALSO AVAILABLE FROM
DANNY AND DRAGON DOOR:

Next Level Strength—The Ultimate Rings and Parallettes Program (2019)

Get Strong—The Ultimate 16 Week Transformation Program (2017)

Street Workout—A Worldwide Anthology of Urban Calisthenics (2016)

Strength Rules—How to Get Stronger Than Almost Anyone (2015)

Diamond-Cut Abs—Minimalist Methods for Maximal Results (2014)

Everybody Needs Training—Proven Success Secrets for the Professional Fitness Trainer (2013)

INDEX OF EXERCISES